# The
# Paradox
## Of
## Modern - Day
# Parenting.

**JANE AND PAUL GAKUYA.**

A
Jane Paul Gakuya Publication.

**Published by**

CREATIONS

+254 724657794

*For more information, contact:*
**Jane and Paul Gakuya**
**P.O BOX 1137-00217, Limuru, Kenya**

Phone: +254 723884931
Email: janewangare9@gmail.com

Phone: +254 702658251
Email: kpaulgakuya@gmail.com

ISBN
979-8332-8403-4-0

# Dedication.

To every parent who desires to raise a Godly generation that will be different in this modern world and become a transgenerational blessing. Also, to every child who wants to rise above parental defects and become successful in life.

# Acknowledgments

To God, our Father, for this excellent assignment toward family reconciliation.

To our spiritual authority **Bishop David O. Oyedep**o – president living faith church worldwide.

Thank you for the insightful and inspiring sermon that enlightened our minds provoking us to live our faith in practical ways indeed we are the testament of the liberation mandate.

**Pastor Boniface Amani Gichina**–Pax mediator international. Your caring and empathetic nature make you an invaluable source of comfort to us always encouraging us during challenging times. Tell Mama we are grateful for opening her home to Paul and giving him the lesson to admire marriage.

**Pastor Park family** –Mission of Mercy International
Thank you for allowing us to work in youth ministry for ten years, and also entrusting us with many charitable programs like feeding programs in school. Helping the single parents in Limuru Kenya and Paying the school fee for thousands of Kenyan children.

We are grateful for the impact you have made and the legacy left in us, your kindness has not gone unnoticed.

To our beautiful daughters **Millie, Alisha**, and **Anaya**. We desire to raise you as Godly children who will become world changers during your generation.

Special thanks to our biological parents **Mr.** and **Mrs. Rev. John Kabugi, Miss Virginia Mwihaki,** and our grandmother **Mrs. Jane Wangari.** Without your unconditional support and modeling, this book never would have come to be. Through your upbringing, your incredible guidance, your care for the people around you, and your devotion in Christ-like inspired us to shed light to the world on kingdom parenting. The struggles and challenges we have seen you fight and overcome created a conquering spirit in us. You are our true heroes.

We appreciate **Mr.** and **Mrs. Joseph Muigai Karanja** for being pillars in our lives. You selflessly supported our wedding ceremony, paid for Jane's University Education, mentored us, and gave us opportunities to grow our careers. Your confidence and support have inspired us to conquer beyond every limitation. All through we know we have a shoulder to lean on. We are heavily indebted.

# TABLE OF CONTENTS.

# Foreword

In the pages that flow forth from "**The Paradox of Modern-Day Parenting,**" readers find a profound exploration of one of today's most vital fields of interest: the multifaceted realm of parenting.

The book, co-authored by Pastor Paul Gakuya and his wife, Jane Paul Gakuya, delves into the challenges and victories associated with raising children in our complex, ever-evolving society.

Pastor Paul and Jane exploit their extensive experiences as parents, as well as their deep spiritual insights, to examine the seismic shifts in societal ethos, norms, and values that have redefined what it means to nurture a child in the modern world. This book is designed to act not just as a guide, but as a companion and a reflective tool for every parent who seeks to understand the implications of parenting in today's world.

Across the sweep of twelve engaging chapters, the authors address pressing questions and prevalent challenges that modern parents face. From understanding the dimensional crises in current parenting models in a chapter titled "Why Modern Parenting is in Crisis," to navigating the critical task of shaping young boys into men of integrity and respect in a chapter titled, "How to Raise Boys to Become Real Men,". The subjects tackled in this book are both timeless and timely.

Pastor Paul and Jane do not shy away from discussing the "Mistakes Parents Commit against Their Children," encouraging a path of awareness and correction that many will find indispensable.

What makes this book unique is its approach that blends practical advice with pastoral wisdom, offering solutions that resonate with the spiritual, emotional, and intellectual needs of modern-day parenting.

The Gakuya's have crafted each chapter to be both insightful and accessible, ensuring that every reader, whether new to parenting or well-versed in the trials and tribulations of family life, finds valuable lessons and encouragement within these pages.

As you embark on this enlightening journey through this book, "The Paradox of Modern-Day Parenting," embrace the opportunity to reflect, learn, and grow. Allow Pastor Paul and Jane to guide you through the quagmire of modern-day parenting, supporting you in your endeavor to raise well-rounded, thoughtful, and loving children.

Welcome to a book that promises not just to inform, but to transform.

Pastor Boniface Amani Gichina<br>Pax Mediators International

# Introduction.

*We may not be able to prepare the future for our children, but we can at least prepare our children for the future.*

*- Franklin D. Roosevelt.*

Every farmer pays attention to the quality of their seeds since they determine the harvest. Many successful people today are products of good parenting.

A child is born clean as a plain sheet of paper; whatever is written on it becomes their life. They are like plasticine, soft, and when molded skillfully, they become what God intended them to be in their purpose and destiny.

*Jeremiah 1:5: Before I formed you in the womb I knew you, before you were born I set you apart, I appointed you as a prophet to the nations."*

The family is the primary source of socialization and the key to every child's development. The truth is that every thief, murderer, fornicator, and rapist emerge from home, and so is every pastor, business person, doctor, engineer, etc. Why diversity? The bringing up, influence, and environment.

> *The family is the primary source of socialization and, hence key to every child's development.*

The systems we were taught by our parents consciously or unconsciously became part of us. If you see any organized and clean woman, it's evident that her mother taught her. Parenting influences all aspects of child development, including social, mental, emotional, and physical. For example, children brought up in a warm, nurturing environment with clear set rules have the best outcome since they grow up possessing high self-esteem, a sense of security, direction, and confidence and, therefore, have high chances of actualizing their dreams, and vice versa.

Parenting in the 21st century has changed and has become challenging due to technological advances, cultural dynamics, and changes in family structure. This has birthed a more informed generation who don't only respond to fear-based parenting but also modern soft parenting approaches. This has resulted in an endangered generation with no morals and values requiring urgent rescue.

Why do we have a very evil generation with decayed or no morals at all? A generation that was prophesied in;

*2 Timothy 3:1-5 This also knows that in the last days, perilous times shall come. For men shall be lovers of their own selves, covetous, boasters, proud, blasphemers, disobedient to parents, unthankful, unholy, without natural affection, trucebreakers, false accusers, incontinent, fierce, despisers of those that are good, Traitors, heady, high minded, lovers of pleasures more than lovers of God; Having a form of godliness, but denying the power thereof: from such turn away* has emerged.

Haven't we heard of all these cases of bitter children, sexual perverts, rebellious, hostile, sinful, proud, and defiant in our society today?  As a result, children's crises have increased, ranging from suicides, teenage parenthood, juvenile criminal activities, identity crises, high rates of mental issues, killings, drug abuse, conflicts, and immature relationships among young people. At an early age, children are struggling with different addictions.

Through various interrogations and interactions with these young people, we have cited parenting as the leading cause of some of these modern problems. And we ask ourselves, where have we gone wrong as parents? God's intention in marriage is to seek a Godly seed. **Malachi 2:15b He** *might seek a godly seed.*

Growing up, we experienced vastly different family dynamics. Jane was raised by her grandmother; alongside her seven aunties, one uncle, and her younger brother who were so instrumental in impacting character in her life and above all introducing her to Jesus. Her single mother worked tirelessly in the city to provide for their basic needs, which were often scarce. The family would sometimes resort to doing manual labour jobs to put food on the table. This upbringing left Jane without a balanced family structure or the fatherly love and guidance that helps shape a child's identity and sense of security.

In contrast, Pastor Paul was fortunate to grow up in a well-balanced family with both of his parents present, despite some challenges. His basic needs were consistently met, and he had a stable home environment.

However, even with these divergent backgrounds, we witnessed first-hand the damaging effects of marital conflict, family disconnection, neglect, divorce, and toxic dynamics within our extended families. These experiences are the exact opposite of what a healthy, functional family should look like. For Jane she believed that marriage is a scam, Paul also wanted to pursue his career, get money and later adopt two daughters.

When we eventually met and married, we found ourselves grappling with a multitude of unanswered questions, gaps, and misconceptions about relationships and parenting. Alarmingly, we also encountered these same issues plaguing the families we counselled through our work in the community and the church.

Determined to find answers and provide solutions, we embarked on an intensive research journey, drawing from our respective expertise in Theology and Psychology.

Through earnest seeking of God's guidance, a deep desire was planted in our hearts to help create healthier families within our community and society at large. We recognized that the path to achieving this starts with addressing the fundamental building block of family life: Parenting.

This book is the culmination of our personal experiences, professional insights, and divine inspiration. By unveiling the paradoxes inherent in modern parenting, we aim to equip readers with the knowledge and tools to navigate the complexities of raising children in today's world and foster thriving, loving, and God-centered families.

# *Chapter 1*

## Crisis in Modern-Day Parenting

*Psalms 127:3 Lo, children are a heritage of the* LORD*: and the fruit of the womb is his reward.*

Parenting in the 21st century has changed. Children are more informed and hence don't respond to the earlier fear-based type of parenting where parents were dictators and harsh, and children adapted without any problem. But today, soft modern approaches have been adopted. God's purpose and objective is for every parent to nurture children as precious gifts from above. Therefore, parenting is a heavenly mandate because he is the giver, as stated in

**James 1: 17:** *Every good gift and every perfect gift is from above...*

A gift is precious and valuable, giving the receiver so much joy upon possession. This is what parenting entails: a joyful journey.

> *This is what parenting entails: a joyful journey;*

But the paradox is, why has parenting become such a problematic affair? Every day, we handle cases of children's rebellion and deviant behavior ranging from drug addiction, peer pressure, fornication, masturbation, lesbianism, etc. What about premature deaths, devil worshipping, and sexual perversion that are being practiced openly by our children? The suicides and mental illnesses, especially among young people?  And the reality is that parents are in mourning and depressed because of their children. What has gone wrong?  Are parents doing their work effectively or contributing to this turmoil?

**Why is parenting challenging in the 21st century?**

**1.     Carnality has led to erosion of Godly morals and values in our society.**

A generation that pushes God away is perishing and foolish.

*Psalms 14:1 The fool hath said there is no God in his heart. They are corrupt; they have done abominable works, none doeth good.*

A generation that has no regard for God has emerged with no Integrity, respect, honesty, Godliness, or righteousness and their actions are evil, not one of them does sound.

They constantly and earnestly defend what is evil to suit their lifestyle.

*Proverbs 14:9 Fools make a mock at sin...*

This has been attributed to the lack of intact Christian teachings and role models from home. Often, we see fathers mandated to be family priests dropping off their wives and children at church and driving off to the bar. Notably, many children come to church alone, leaving their parents at home.

Parents do not teach children about God through devotion, word, worship, or prayer time. The truth is that it begins with the parents. Do you know God? If yes, introduce him to the children from a young age. God's command to the parents is to impress God's precept on their minds and penetrate their hearts with the truth, which is the foundation of their Christian journey. **John 3:32.** *Then you will know the truth, and the truth will set you free.* "Do you find yourself struggling with prayer before eating or sleeping? Yes, it's simply because your parents never taught you.  To preserve this generation, we need to instill Godly values through the meditation of scriptures and training on how to pray, worship, and teach these from our homes.

We are privileged to serve the youth and often discuss real-life issues affecting them. A 17-year-old boy confessed that he is glued to drug addiction but secretly.  He learned it from his role model, his father. The mother sometimes attends church but has never discovered the truth. He says that they have never had a family devotion at home. He only knew Jesus in Sunday school. But by the grace of God, he was delivered from that siege forever.

Carnality gives the devil the legal ground to torment our children and destroy their destinies.

In **Deuteronomy 28:28**, God pronounced curses upon a disobedient generation through madness, confusion, and blindness, which is evident today.

> *Carnality gives the devil a legal ground to torment our children and destroy their destinies*

Vs 41 states that parents will raise sons and daughters, but they will be taken to the captivity of the world since the promotion of the wicked is from shame to shame. **Proverbs 3:35**

Research shows that children emerging from homes where parents take responsibility for teaching Christian morals are less deviant behavior compared to Christian homes where parents are busy and don't create time to teach Christian morals. God regulates and kills physical appetites. No spirit of addiction, sexual perversion, or rebellion can survive in a spiritual home saturated with Christian teachings and prayers. Just visit an environment like a university; why are some students in bars partying and dancing half naked with men while others are sitting in an auditorium for Christian union? Those students experienced different parenting. It only takes the hand of God to save this generation through us by planting a seed of God in their hearts.

## 2.	Parenting in the digital era.

We are living in a technologically advanced world. Exposure to a lot of information that is easily accessible has led to a more informed generation. The effects of television, computers, and phones are evident, especially on social media platforms. At the early age of four years, a child can operate a smartphone/tablet independently without parental assistance. Children have become cartoon addicts which tamper with their belief systems by creating a world of fantasy rather than reality. Some of these cartoons and games have romantic scenes, which are platforms the devil is using to instill the spirit of lust in the minds of our children and young people. Jane encountered a boy of seven years who had been battling pornography addiction which was instilled by cartoons and the desire craved for watching real porn.

Explicit pornographic content in songs, dressing modes, and movies has corrupted the mindsets of young people. For example, every trending video or song has sexual content, indecent dressing, and sexual dancing styles, which encourage perverse sexual practices such as; fornication, masturbation, lesbianism, bestiality, rape, etc.

These practices open the doors for spiritual attacks that torment the destiny of our children. A youth confessed to having slept with over fifty men, including relatives. She says she lacks the power to control sexual urges or lust. This spirit came due to the pornographic content she watched on her phone.  Slowly, she slipped into sex addiction. Whenever you awaken love at the wrong age, it becomes problematic automatically.

*Songs of Solomon 8:4 I charge you, O daughters of Jerusalem, that ye stir not up, nor awake my love, until he please.*

**Social Media is a dragon;** Social media platforms normalize sex, which has become a tool to enrich themselves, especially to get a job or any favor. Today, many young girls believe that

*Social Media is a dragon*

having an old man, "mubabaz," as a lover is typical to have a lavish life like what social media portrays, even at the expense of destroying other people's marriages. This has contributed to so many young girls trading their precious season with sex for money. The information watched on digital gadgets creates curiosity among young people; hence, they go to practice. The Bible in;

*2 Timothy 2:22, Flee also youthful lusts: but follow righteousness, faith, charity, and peace with them, calling on the Lord out of a pure heart.*

The Bible admonishes young people to flee from sexual evil desires. Pornography and masturbation have become the order of the day and, as a result, lead to crises like teenage pregnancy and abortions.

**Genesis 39:1-8** highlights the case of Joseph, who shuns the sexual desires of Potiphar's wife. Today, girls sleep with bosses and other people's husbands to get money and other favors. Where is the Joseph and Daniel generation who stood with the truth of God? This is what is swallowing the future and the destiny of our children.

The sad part is that parents have also become phone addicts, leaving no time to interact with their children. Also, phones have contributed to rising cases of divorces and conflicts. Let's minimize children's exposure to the internet;

today, even a kindergarten child has a phone. How? This is what is destroying the minds and attitudes of our children.

We advise watching television and programs under parental control or permanently removed. The Internet has also become a recruiting platform for LGBTQ, militia groups, occult groups, etc. There are over 4.2 million pornographic sites on the internet and many lesbian/ gay recruitment sites. But if social media can be used positively, it is a source of positive information that can assist in molding their destinies.

**3.      Life priorities have changed.**
Balancing family, career, education, business, and parenting has become challenging. In earlier times, women were especially homemakers, which gave them time to raise their children well. Women today are career-oriented; after maternity leave, a child at three months is left under the care of a nanny. Parenting has become a matter of delegation to other people.

Today, priority is given to making money and acquiring wealth.

*In Mathew 6:24: No man can serve two masters: for either he will hate the one, and love the other, or else he will hold to the one, and despise the other. Ye cannot serve God and mammon.*

It admonishes us against an undue devotion to money. We don't refute the idea that money is necessary, but it should not be a priority over your children. We see parents leaving early in the morning, and upon returning at night, children are asleep. This has broken the bond and emotional attachment with the children, just like as many have confessed.

One time, Jane was working with the County Government and used to travel very far, while Pst. Paul served in a mission church. Therefore, she left the house at 6 am when our children were asleep and would return at 7 pm. After some time, our daughter would cry once her mother pick her up; she couldn't feed her, touch her, bathe her, or sleep with her. To make matters worse, she began calling her nanny's mum.  We realized her mother was losing connection. She immediately took a leave of 4 months, and we laid off the house girl to look after our children, which was not easy. After the break, she returned with a resignation letter and started a business to look after our children. Things changed, the attachment was restored, and we became fulfilled. She got the time to train and instill upright character as we desired.

Parents, no matter your position in your workplace, your family will be all you have after retirement. The time and sacrifice you invest in them will determine how they will handle and treat you after retirement. Don't substitute them with anything. Parenting has no breaks or leaves. It's a continuous process. Therefore, parents should strike a balance. Today, parenting is driven by provision creating **responsibility attachment** at the expense of emotional attachment. This has caused chaos because children lack that sense of love and belonging.  They mess up their destinies while looking for love to fill the void. God intends for the family to dwell in love, unity, and oneness so that he can command a blessing.

*Psalms 133:1How good and pleasant it is **when** God's people live together in unity!*

**NOTE**. Children Require Presence more than presents!

> *Children require more Presence than presents.*

## 4.     Change of family institution and family structure.

Many new family structures have emerged today, such as single parenthood, neglectful parenting, extended family parenting, blended family, etc. Children are raised by single mothers/fathers, absentee fathers, stepmothers/fathers, grandparents, children's homes, etc. This has created an unbalanced way of parenting. A child should be raised by a balanced father and mother family to have the same principles. A child confessed to being raised by three different families at once. By the biological mother and stepfather; other times, he visits the biological father, stepmother, and grandparents during holidays. This has confused him since all parties have different rules and principles.

The rising cases of divorces and marital conflicts have contributed to a rise of more family structures like co-parenting, where a child is brought up by parents who live separately. These children are exposed to confusion and modeled in between crises.

Decreased number of children within a family; Families then were large, with 8 and 9 children being the least born within a family. Parents could balance all their needs since everyone would fight to get their space, including food, love, and belonging. Today, families are smaller with 1 to 2 children, and parents grant them all the love, attention, good schools, and good life to the point of over-spoiling them. That's why some feel their siblings are favored over them, creating issues of love deficiency, insecurity, low resilience, and low self-acceptance.

Other matters like polygamy sets children to confusion about the correct format of a family. Many tend to become polygamous in the future due to family influence, which is against the will of God, as stated in **Genesis 2:22-24,** creating more crisis.

## 5.    Evil and insecure world changing the patterns of parenting.

We are living in a dangerous, insecure world where parenting has been left to the immediate family. Earlier parenting was easy since a child belonged to the whole community. Today, entrusting your children, even to relatives, has become extremely difficult. We have dealt with over hundred cases of child molestation, rape, and sodomy from relatives, uncles, stepfathers, etc.

A girl confessed to having been raped severally by her birth father at the tender age of nine years. All through her high school, the rape continued, and upon confiding to her mother, she ruthlessly beat her, claiming she was lying against her father to destroy their marriage. Severally, she conceived, but she had to abort four times. After twelve years, this girl finds out that she is HIV positive, her uterus is damaged completely, and she can't bear children all her life. This situation threw her into depression, and upon meeting her, she was in hospital due to a failed suicide; this is the world we are living in now.

The majority of cases that my wife and I have handled emanate from sexual harassment; children being used for ritual purposes and witchcraft. You are the only safe ground they have. Be watchful even with the house managers, shamba boys, neighbors, teachers, and relatives. In case of any behavior change exhibited by your children, be quick to find out and take necessary measures.

The Bible highlights the times we are living in now;

*In Mathew 10:21And the brother shall deliver up the brother to death, and the father the child: and the children shall rise up against their parents, and cause them to be put to death.*

*In Genesis 19:35 – 36.* Highlights a story of Lots daughters who intoxicated their father with wine and slept with him. They gave birth to a cursed generation of Moabites and Ammonites who all fought with the Israelites, God's chosen generation.

The truth is that despite changes in parenting dynamics, the foundation of God's word cannot be substituted. It stands as the sure and only way of parenting.

*2 Timothy 2:19 -Nevertheless the foundation of God standeth sure, having this seal...*

6.     **Loss of culture and adoption of Western culture.**
Brian Howell and Janelle Paris define culture as the total way of life. Everything we learn after being born into the world enables us to function effectively. The culture a child lives in contributes to a set of values, customs shared assumptions, and ways of living that influence development throughout

the lifespan. Every Community has its culture, standards, and codes of conduct that determine how people live and treat one another, the behaviors it upholds, food consumed, language, way of dressing, etc. We are each carefully indoctrinated from birth in the pattern of behavior that adults around us consider appropriate. By becoming aware of what's happening, we have already been pressed into the cultural mode.

God created humans as individuals with a culture-producing mandate. The Bible is not against culture because Jesus himself was submissive and incarnated into the Jewish culture of Nazareth. But every scripture is meant to confront us and bring a new way of thinking.

*2 Timothy 3:16 All Scripture is God-breathed and is useful for teaching, rebuking, correcting, and training in righteousness.*

Therefore, every culture that contradicts and exalts a harmful demonic lifestyle is against what God would have men practice, as stated in;

> *A culture that contradicts and exalts a harmful demonic lifestyle is against what God would have men practice.*

*Mark 7:13: Making the word of God of no effect through your tradition, which ye have delivered: and many such things do ye.*

Today, however, incorporating Western cultures has hugely influenced parenting since they influence their belief, thinking, identity, and value systems. For instance, Interactions among different communities have brought about the exchange of cultural practices. Today, we see children having identity crises; they don't know who they are or where they belong, and that's why many have resolved to be lesbians and homosexuals, even in African countries. This is because they have copied what others are practicing. They even have their activists who fight for their rights. This is an abomination and against the standards of God. **Ephesians 5:3-5**

The African culture, where we had older men and women to help teach children morals and values, is no longer present. If you look closely at the mode of dressing, the language, weird behaviors, and celebrations exhibited by children today, you would conclude that we need help. This shows that the outer defective world has overpowered home training.

Who is there to teach our girls and boys the traditions and cultural values of our community? Who is teaching women to be respectful and submissive wives in homes? Who is teaching men to become responsible fathers and husbands? That's why we are raising half-baked men and women who have no regard for family values and dignity. How can a real man marry and live in the lady's house in the name of love? How can a man go and sleep in their in-law's house? Traditionally, this was unacceptable. What about our girls? How can a girl have sexual intercourse with a father, uncle, or relative? What about immodest dressing, especially in church and in front of the elders and respectable people in society? These issues show a loss of cultural values and traditions.

## 7.    Too busy syndrome.

Today, parents have become so busy looking for money, hence lack time to spend with their children. Children have been left in the care of house managers, boarding schools, daycares, and relatives. And even during school holidays, they are sent upcountry to visit their grandparents. Other parents are working abroad. Money has become a separating factor. Research shows that these children lack parental love and connection. When you are busy, the devil is busy feasting on your children's morals and destiny through television, peer pressure, and young relationships, hence planting an evil mindset and attitude that is messing up their destiny. This has led to behavioral problems, emotional problems, depression, stress, and mental illnesses.

Children do not require much time; research shows that ten minutes of **quality time** per day can mean much more. Take time to connect, bond, and build trust with your children. Go for recreational activities, cook together, play together, etc. Every sacrifice you make will count. As a mum, I remember quitting my employment to raise my children. One could resolve to do a business or work from home to look after one's family, especially mothers. I have seen women holding up their careers and still do intentional parenting. Create a bond with them so that when they face a challenge, they will open up to you...

## 8.	Toxic parenting.

This occurs when parents have unresolved issues within themselves due to marital conflicts, divorces, past relationship disappointments, bitterness, anger and resentment, pressure from loss of jobs, etc. This pressure is directed at the children through physical assault, name-calling, and yelling, and some have been killed. This has resulted in raising bitter children who are even mentally challenged and possess low self-esteem. This, in turn, increases the rate of crime, suicides, fornication, and murder.

We counseled with a lady who killed her child by hitting her against the wall due to anger and bitterness she had incubated for years after a relationship breakup. Many street children confess to us that they run away from home due to abuse. Psychologists say that a child brought up in violence, watching the dad beating the mum, ends up being violent, too.

Do you remember the twenty-two-year-old boy who killed his entire family in Kiambu County? Upon examination, he was declared unfit mentally to stand trial. Upon interrogation, he cited that his parent favored the other siblings over him, which bred anger and resentment, but probably was not the truth. But there was a negative mindset in him already. What had led to this deep grudge to the point of killing his parents and brothers? What of numerous suicides among children? There is a big problem.

*A toxic Parent Creates a Hostile Home Environment.*

A toxic parent creates a hostile home environment; they are abusive, emotionally unstable, and neglectful. They use fear, intimidation, and humiliation as tools to ensure they get compliance from their children. In return, these children grow up with fear, low self-esteem, insecurity issues, anger, bitterness, and resentment, hate themselves, and have mental health issues. When this generation is released to the world, they release negative energy, which has brought about many crises due to parenting.

Therefore, from the reasons discussed above, it's evident that the outside systems of the world are strong enough to affect a child. Thus, it is wise to strengthen home training so that a child will gain the stamina to interact with the outside world without losing home values.

**In Proverbs** *22:6, Train a child in the way he should go: And when he is old, he will not depart from it.*

Here, it means that if no systems are taught diligently, this child will depart and be torn down. The devil will swallow their destiny. Begin from a tender age. The foundation is critical and forms the base of every parenting.

*Psalms 11:3 If the foundations are destroyed, what can the righteous do?*

# *Chapter 2*

## Godly Parenting is a Sure Foundation.

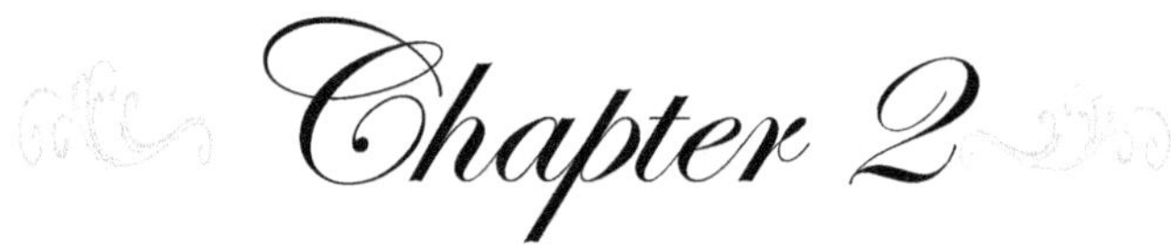


Godly parenting entails raising children according to the principles of the word of God. It's raising them to see themselves through the lenses of their maker. *In Psalms 127:3, children are a heritage and a reward from God.*

Therefore, their creator is the only one who can understand them. In their weaknesses, help and pray for them to become what God intended for their destiny.

Modern Science can be limited. Why? How can you explain the formation of a child in the womb? How can one get seven children at a go? What about testimonies we have heard of conceiving without fallopian tubes, uterus etc.? It can only be God. God never fails, and He is unlimited.

Godly parenting is a heavenly mandate. It's a command from God. God has entrusted his children to us as caretakers, to which I believe we will give an account. When a fish is taken out of the water, it dies immediately. If you disconnect a child from the source – God, the child will grow to fail in life, which is the main problem causing crisis in modern parenting today. Foundation is what roots a child in development. If you lay the wrong foundation, be sure the child will have developmental defects that will show in behavior.

Let's analyze God's objective and expectations regarding parenting.

*In Genesis 1:26 – 28 And, God said, Let us make man in our image, after our likeness: and let them have dominion over the fish of the sea, and over the fowl of the air, and over the cattle, and over all the earth, and over every creeping thing that creepeth upon the earth. So God created man in his image, in the image of God created him; male and female created him them. And God blessed them, and God said unto them, Be fruitful, and multiply, and replenish the earth, and subdue it: and have dominion over the fish of the sea, and over the fowl of the air, and over every living thing that moveth upon the earth.*

From Genesis, God had some expectations for us, which include;

1.         **Fruitfulness and Multiplication**

It's a command to increase in number after His image. Adam and Eve fulfilled the mandate in **Genesis 5:1-3**. God created a man (male) and a woman (man with a womb) and gave them the capability to reproduce. Therefore, it's evident that any case of barrenness is an affliction from the devil since God gave a woman and man the ability to reproduce. Multiplication is the only sure way to preserve generations.

2.     **To pass on the nature and character of GOD to the child.**

**Genesis 1:26**; God created man possessing his DNA; through salvation, we have the nature of God as our father.

*John 1:12 But as many as received him, to them gave the power to become the sons of God, even to them that believe in his name:*

God expects the born-again parents' faith in Christ to be conveyed to their offspring. Being formed in God's image means we possess God's behavior and character. His values, love, and kindness should be passed on to our children.

## 3.    To raise Godly offspring

*Malachi 2:14-15 Yet ye say Wherefore? Because the LORD hath been witness between thee and the wife of thy youth, against whom thou hast dealt treacherously: yet is she thy companion, and the wife of thy covenant. And did not he make one? Yet had he the residue of the spirit. And wherefore one? That he might seek a godly seed. Therefore, take heed to your spirit, and let none deal treacherously against the wife of his youth.*

God's primary objective for parents is to raise a Godly generation who will, in turn, raise another Godly generation, which is a principle in *Joshua 4:6-7*

Do you know why God entrusted Abraham with a generation? Because He knew He would command his house in the ways of the lord– *Genesis 18:19*

Every generation in the bible was traced from a Godly seed. For example, Abraham had a firstborn Ishmael with Hagar **(Genesis 16:15)**, his wife's servant, but God recognized Isaac (covenant child) as the preserver of generation. Ishmael was cursed (Genesis 16:12) – he became the generation of foreign nations who fought with the Israelites, God's chosen race. After battling with the angel, Isaac became the father of Jacob, who was named Israel. Therefore, parenting is a ministry; we are custodians and caretakers in partnership with God to raise a generation of God. The big question is, are you worthy of trust?

> *Parenting is a Ministry.*

**Six Fundamental truths about GODLY parenting.**

**1.      Children are fruits and blessings of a marriage covenant.**

God gave the marriage ordinance before speaking the blessing of children. He knew a child should be raised in a stable home environment of mother and father. Cain, Abel, and Seth were the first children born after the fall of man. *Genesis 4:1-2.* Isaac was a product of Abraham and Sarah. Samuel Hannah and Elkanah.

Are we saying that a couple that marries right cannot lack children? It simply means bareness is not God's idea. It is a war in which the couple should pray to get the fruit of the womb.

What about the fate of children born out of wedlock; fornication and adultery?

In Genesis *21:8-9*, we see God disregarding Ishmael, the son of Abraham, and Hagar, the mistress, and regards Isaac as the sole heir.

Also in *Genesis 25:5-6. Abraham gave all he had to Isaac and gave gifts to the sons of the concubines and sent them away.*

Also, the case of Bathsheba, Uriah's wife, and King David in **2 Samuel 12:13-25** whom God died as a result of punishment for the sin he committed. David's house was cursed with the sword; others took his wives. **2 Samuel 13** records Incest and rape in the family bloodline when Absalom raped his sister Tamar. David had done evil in the sight of the Lord. God had to send Nathan to David to reveal his anger toward him. Was God not merciful to kill? The bottom line is these children are born under a spiritual fight. Under the Mosaic Law, breaking this covenant in the Old Testament brought about punishment until the 10th generation.

*Deuteronomy 23:2 No one born of a forbidden union may enter the assembly of the Lord. Even to the tenth generation, none of his descendants may enter the assembly of the Lord.*

Also, these children grow up with social problems and defects. Many are raised by their mothers, absent fathers, grandparents, and relatives. This, in most cases, has caused abuse and negligence among these children in their upbringing. Many have missed basic needs like food, education, love, identity, guidance, and attachment which in turn has breaded a bitter, unbalanced, and emotionally crippled generation.

How do you explain a case where a man can leave his family and children and remarry without taking care of his blood? The probability is that this man was never raised in a balanced family and was never taught to understand the value of wholesome fatherhood. This is the cause of single parenthood today, where women are left struggling with their children for their source of livelihood.  It's an era of absentee fathers who are always in drinking and entertainment joints, abandoning their children. But the bigger picture is the plan of the devil to finish the generation by corrupting the seed (fathers).

*Galatians 6:8 For he that soweth to his flesh shall of the flesh reap corruption; but he that soweth to the Spirit shall of the Spirit reap life everlasting.*

In most instances, this can evoke generational curses upon the family bloodline. In our line of work, many mothers have confessed that they can trace a generational chain in their families where certain people get children out of wedlock, mostly the firstborns.

But through the blood of Jesus, we are saved; therefore, these children must fight a war to win against singlehood.

*Galatians 3:13 Christ hath redeemed us from the curse of the law, being made a curse for us: for it is written, cursed is everyone that hangeth on a tree:*

2.      **God owns our children.**

*Psalms 127:3. Lo, children are a heritage of the LORD: and the fruit of the womb is his reward.*

They are gifts from above and a blessing to the family. No one can give themself a child; it's a reward from God. Gifts are highly valued and received with thanks. Gifts are priceless and perfect.

*James 1:17 Every good and perfect gift is from above...*

Take every child as a gift regardless of their weaknesses, value and treasure them by training them in the lord's ways. To preserve the future generation, we must raise Christian giants who will carry on the legacy of raising Godly children, and the surest foundation is giving Jesus to them.

Whatever you treasure, you will, without a doubt, place a premium value on. If you mistreat or neglect children, especially in our modern days, God, who is their father, will deal with you. Nothing in your life shall prosper. The tears of pain from a child reach to his Heavenly Father – God. Be a blessing to them, and God will reward you for your obedience.

**3.      It's a command from God. Parenting is a Heavenly order or law from above, not an earthly mandate.**

Deuteronomy 6:6-6: God commands us to always be diligent in parenting. *"When thou sittest in the house, walking and lying too."* Let the word of God be the first and the last thing they hear when they sleep.  The promises and commands of God do not add sorrow since, in the end, they are rewarding. (**1 John 5:3. Hebrews 10:36**)

The bible narrates a story of King Lemuel, whose mother's teachings stood out.

Proverbs 31:1 King Lemuel's words, the prophecy *his mother taught him. What, my son? And what, the son of my womb? and what, the son of my vows?³ Give not thy strength unto women, nor thy ways to that which destroyeth kings. It is not for kings, O Lemuel, it is not for kings to drink wine; nor for Princes strong drink:*

Every teaching is beneficial in the lives of our children.

Refusal to train your children in the fear of God is disobedience, which breeds shame and reproach as consequences.

*Deuteronomy 28:15 it shall come to pass, if thou wilt not hearken unto the voice of the Lord thy God, to observe to do all his commandments and his statutes which I command thee this day; that all these curses shall come upon thee, and overtake thee*

How many children are causing pain in the lives of their parents?  If you sleep on the assignment, the devil will plant an evil seed in your children, which will cause pain, regrets, and depression in you as a parent, and also, God will reject your children.

*1Samuel 15:23says that rebellion is the sin of witchcraft, and stubbornness is iniquity and idolatry. Because thou hast rejected the word of the Lord, he hath also rejected thee from being king.*

And after you have done the will of God, you will see the fruits of your labor- Hebrews 10:36.

4.      Children are like arrows in the hand of a mighty man.

*Psalms 127:4-5 As arrows are in the hand of a mighty man; so are children of the youth. Happy is the man that hath his quiver full of them: they shall not be ashamed but speak with the enemies in the gate.*

Arrows are lethal weapons of war. Children are defenders, protectors, and security of their parents.  We remember our uncle fighting a man who abused his mother. They will defend you during calamities, want, and need. They are a source of support and cover. They will protect you from enemies like poverty, lack, and weakness. Recently, my husband and I embarked on a blessed journey of building a beautiful Stoney house for my mother, who was living in a small iron sheet house. And God gave us this revelation that poverty is an enemy.

**Verse 5**. They stop the works of the devil.  Our responsibility is to fashion them to be obedient to their call. We often admire Bishop David Oyedepo's (Founder of Living Faith International) children, spiritual giants working in the kingdom of God and bringing down all the devil's works just as their father and mother.  This is a result of Godly parenting. The same grace shall be replicated in you in Jesus' name.

5.      **Children are good seeds.**

*Mathew 13:38 The field is the world; the good seed are the children of the kingdom; but the tares are the children of the wicked one;*

Every farmer pays attention to the quality of seeds since they determine harvest. Kingdom parenting guarantees labor with profit. The word of God is the seed; a child's heart represents the good ground bearing a precious gift, but when it grows, it is larger than the garden.

*Mathew 13:32 Which indeed is the least of all seeds: but when it is grown, it is the greatest among herbs, and becometh a tree, so the birds of the air come and lodge in the branches thereof.*

This signifies an impact on the children that is beneficial to everyone.

In **Jeremiah35:5-6** Jonadab ordered his family not to drink wine, which was evident when wine was presented and they refused to drink. Also, in **2 Timothy 1:5**, Timothy's faith was passed by Eunice, his mother, and Loise, his grandmother.

Therefore, plant quality seeds and be sure of a bumper harvest. Don't allow the enemy to sow tares in the hearts of your children.

*Mathew 13:25 But while men slept, his enemy came and sowed tares among the wheat, and went his way.*

God will establish your seed forever in Jesus' name.

*Psalms 89:4 Thy seed will I establish forever, and build up thy throne to all generations.*

## 6.      Parenting is not a funfair but a warfare.

Parenting is challenging since the devil plans to destroy their destiny to eliminate generations. This is evident today with the rising cases of barrenness, premature deaths, rates of suicides and abuses among children.

*John 10:10 The thief cometh not, but for to steal, kill, and destroy: I am come that they might have life and have it more abundantly.*

We need not to be ignorant of the schemes the devil is using to destroy them as *2 Corinthians 2:11 states that lest Satan should get an advantage of us: for we are not ignorant of his device.* It means we should be armed spiritually and mentally to know the alternatives and shortcuts he uses to challenge the word of God. *Ephesians 6:11 Put on the whole armor of God that ye may be able to stand against the wiles of the devil.* It also requires us to train our children on weapons of war to guard themselves because the son of God was manifested to destroy the works of the devil *1 John 3:8*

In the bible, 'covenant' women had issues with bareness, but God blessed them with covenant children. Sarah and Abraham begot Isaac. Hannah and Elkanah, who begot Prophet Samuel, the greatest prophet of that time. Therefore, as a parent, you must be heavily armed to fight against enemies of your children's destinies. We wrestle against the principalities and power of darkness that are determined to destroy our generations. - *Ephesians 6:1*

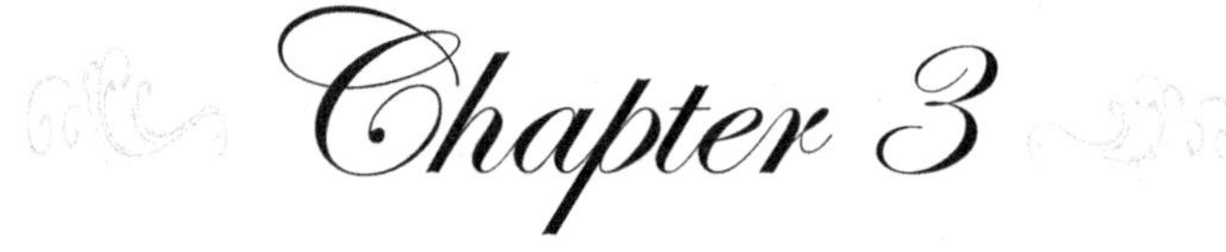

# Chapter 3

## The Stages/Levels of Parenting.

As children develop in every aspect, they learn new things that influence their behavior. Therefore, parenting should vary depending on the age of the child, the nature of the child, the environment, and milestone development. Parenting styles should vary; raising a teenager differs from raising a child and an adult. The problem parents exhibit is applying the same parenting mode throughout a child's development, creating more crises.

We see Jesus as a perfect example of growth in levels, which implies mental and physical development, as well as in his assignment.

*Luke 2:52 and Jesus increased in wisdom, stature, and favor with God and man.*

Let us briefly analyze every stage of development and offer tips on the best parenting strategy to ensure your child grows well.

## STAGE 1

**Conception To 9 Months**

The first conception of a baby happens in the mind of God. *Jeremiah 1:5 "Before I formed you in the womb I knew you, before you were born, I set you apart; I appointed you as a prophet to the nations."* this means that the destiny of our children is already conceived in the mind of God even before they are born.

Therefore, the foundation of parenting begins from the womb. Conception is where we shape and agree on the destiny of a child by faith based on our revelation of what God has said concerning them. *Luke 1:45 and blessed is she that believed, for there shall be a performance of those things which were told to her from the lord.* Begin to shape the destiny of your children right from the womb. Physically give the child the right atmosphere to grow well; eat a balanced diet, take enough rest, avoid heavy duties, go to antenatal clinics, and avoid alcohol and caffeine use.

Spiritually, set the atmosphere by confessing and prophesying the word of God for them. It is proven that a child can understand sounds outside the mother's body.

**And it happened, when Elizabeth heard the greeting of Mary, that the babe leaped in her womb; and Elizabeth was filled with the Holy Spirit. *Luke 1:41.***

Confess what you desire your child to become. Declare that they shall be a sign and wonder **(Isaiah 8:18)**, they will always be the head and not the tail **(Deuteronomy 28: 13)**, you shall grow in wisdom and stature, in favor with God and men **(Luke 2; 52)**, the spirit of excellence dwell in you **(Daniel 6; 3)**. The right spiritual atmosphere clears every block set against the child and ensures their destiny is fulfilled at ease.

This has worked for our children; whatever we confess manifests in their lives. In our marriage, we experienced two miscarriages, but by God's grace, we conceived again. During the fourth month, the devil struck again, and my wife began to bleed; together we declared life upon the child, upon arrival in the hospital for a scan, the baby was alive.

Throughout the pregnancy, declaration became our lifestyle; by God's grace, we gloriously welcomed our third born, who was so healthy and weighty. we have seen my children grow without struggle, favored by men, and people compete to pay for their school fees and buy goodies like shoes and clothes.

Beware that the devil is never happy with the fruit of the womb and often tries to eliminate the seed at all costs. Miscarriages and stillbirths are the works of the enemy. Wage war spiritually against his works.

Pregnancy is warfare; when a child is born, give them a name that has a Godly meaning and purpose. The destiny of a child can be determined at childbirth.

*I Chronicles 4:9-10: Jabez was more honorable than his brothers. His mother had named him Jabez, saying, "I gave birth to him in pain."*

The name carries the mission, purpose, and destiny. For example, Jesus means savior because his assignment was to save humanity from the penalty of sin. When God wanted to change the destiny of his people in the bible, he concentrated on changing their names. Example: Abram to Abraham, Sarai to Sarah, and Jacob to Israel.

We have heard many people confessing to having suffered because of being named after their kin, and they end up possessing the same traits they possess.
Let the child be dedicated and blessed by a spiritual authority like Samuel. In **1 Samuel 1:27-28, I prayed for this**

child, and the Lord *granted me what I asked of him. So now I give him to the LORD. For his whole life, he will be given over to the LORD." And he worshiped the LORD there.* This seals the covenant of blessings and establishes a Godly atmosphere in their lives for a great start. After that, do not drop the ball. Keep on nurturing the child in the ways of the Lord.

## STAGE 2
### Parenting Toddlers from Age 1 – 5 Years.

> *A tender tree is easier to straighten than when it overgrows.*

A tender tree is easier to straighten than when it overgrows. – *African Proverb.*

This is the primary and best foundation stage of parenting. At this level, the parent practices an art known as '**loving discipline.**' The child has developed activities, including listening, reading, and playing with friends. They are learning to do things independently, even without considering the dangers.

Children will ask questions out of curiosity, seeking answers. As a parent, your answer forms the fundamental truth for the child. They are also prone to show intense emotional tantrums, which, as a parent, calmness will shape their emotional intelligence. Children handle pressure by observing how you handle your pressure towards them.

Children learn through observation, listening, exploring, experimenting, and questioning.

At four years old, a child is in kindergarten and has access to other children with different behaviors. Ensure you consistently have established moral and behavioral systems that they will follow. Even if they encounter different systems, unlearning the training received at home will be difficult. Develop a culture of playing, study, neatness, personal grooming, good manners, wholesome language, respect for themselves and others, praying, singing, and reciting short memory verses to widen their mental capacity.

Sometimes, children want to engage in forceful and risky behaviors that parents know can cause harm—for example, playing in a bucket of water, playing with fire, or sliding on a slippery floor. Here, we use '**Control or policeman**' parenting because their mental capacity is too young to reason that the behavior is dangerous.

Generally, instill discipline by light caning or pinching, withdraw some privileges they love most, reward them when they exhibit positive behavior, offer affirmation, and convey love and respect to engender a sense of security. Ensure you draw boundaries but in love. The purpose is to teach and correct what seemed difficult at that time.

*Hebrews 12:10-11.  No discipline seems pleasant at the time but painful. Later, it produces a harvest of righteousness and peace for those trained by it.*

The issue of disciplining has been widely misunderstood and misinterpreted in modern times; we often see children being abused physically in the name of correction. The Bible talks of not sparing the rod but implies applying the spiritual rod as a discipline tool.

*Important Note:* *Children learn better when taught how to behave well instead of being scolded for misbehaving.*

*Children learn better when taught how to behave well instead of being scolded for misbehaving.*

## STAGE 3

### AGE 5 TO 12 YEARS –TRAINING.

Having already laid a good foundation on right and wrong, introduce a system check that ensures every discipline and behavior is followed. Pay attention to their ability to follow directions. At this age, every behavior you desire to impact in your child must be built at this stage. The child is growing physically, spiritually, socially, emotionally, and mentally, and therefore, more programs to help in this growth should be introduced at this stage.

For example, physical activities, behavior change, good communication skills, confidence, personal grooming, neatness, good manners, cultivating their own opinions, managing their allowances, relationships with other people, and so on.

Training should be tailor-made based on the **nature of the child**. This is because children possess different temperaments and personalities. Some are passive or quiet, active and very loud. **Active children** are results and action-oriented. They are self-motivated and cooperative when assigned a particular task. They are always curious to know what's next.

Therefore, assigning them duties will make them more effective and self-driven; otherwise, they will go out of control and domineer without parental structure. These children are natural leaders, so extra effort is required to nurture them. This child possesses a very high inborn self-esteem. As a parent, please don't kill it; nurture it because these children are annoyance sometimes. Expose them to leadership platforms at their level, like leading songs in church or reciting a poem before people. The danger comes once they face ridicule and criticism. They tend to lower their esteem, and the child dies off slowly.

**The passive,** quiet, and sensitive children are less active and dramatic and are more attached to their feelings. They seek attention, empathy, and validation for their actions. They respond to encouragement more than being pushed. They are good followers once assigned a task; they follow but can't go beyond. They thrive in a quiet environment of peace and calmness. For such kids, train them, but don't over-push them beyond their capability because it will lower their esteem. Therefore, with this in mind, it will assist you in dealing with a child as per their nature and also cease comparing your children.

The Bible gives us an example of Jesus In *Luke 2:46-52;* when Jesus was 12 years old, when they attended the annual Passover feast with their parents in Jerusalem, he remained behind only to be found in the temple listening to the teachings from the teachers of laws. At this age, he had the understanding and wisdom about his father's business, as stated in Luke 2: 52. *Jesus increased in wisdom and stature and favor with God and men.*

**Here are some suggested ideas to achieve this milestone.**
- Have a timetable of events per day. Wake up time, time to watch cartoons, playing time, school time.
- Hold spiritual programs; Prayer at mealtimes, worship together, read the word of God, go to church, and encourage them to serve in the children's church department.
- Assign tasks at home, including cleaning utensils and the house and arranging their bedroom.

- On money matters, assist them in budgeting, offering in church, cultivating their saving culture by opening an account, and ensuring they save in a bank or saving box. Buy goodies using a small portion of their money.

- Buy story books to cultivate their reading culture and widen their mental capacity and reasoning. Have them recite small poems and memory verses.

- Assist in controlling their outside influence by assisting them to choose the best peers and friends who will positively impact them.

- Spend time with them in outings and outdoor activities. This cements your bond as a family.

- Let them know the expectations, Dos, and DONTs of the family.

The purpose is to train and nurture them in the love of God so that, despite outside influences, they will not lose home training. **Ephesians 6-4, Mathew 22:37-39.** By the age of 12 years, the child should be firm, disciplined, confident, well-behaved, respectful, and well-packaged with the best values.

> *Any Behavior Not Instilled at This Age will be Difficult to Format later in Life.*

Important Note: *Any Behavior Not Instilled at This Age Will Be Difficult to Format later in life.*

## STAGE 4

## RAISING TEENAGERS 13-18 YEARS.

This is the adolescent age, believed to be the most challenging level of parenting. This is the level where many teenage boys and girls divert their God-ordained destinies by engaging in risky behavior like drug abuse, sexual perversion, peer influence, crime, and gangs leading to addictions.

Most lose their focus lose their destinies, and others have died early, burying unfulfilled potential and dreams to the grave. This is an age of realization where they develop their values, priorities, and goals and gain a sense of belonging to a community and the world around them. They love being recognized and guided and seek their parents' and peers' attention.

On the other hand, parents are full of uncertainties and insecurities and want to protect their children against mistakes, bad choices, and influences. They are torn between whether they are becoming too involved in their teen's life or under-involved. Parenting becomes hard when parents remain rigid and don't change their parenting style. Teenagers are grown and can reason at this age, but not entirely. As a parent, the knowledge to understand what is going on in their lives will assist you in offering relevant information.

**Noticeable Behaviours Teenagers Exhibit**

**a.** They experience a lot of body and hormonal changes, which trigger changes in sexual appetite, opposite-sex attraction, and emotional outbursts.

As a parent, be stable emotionally and put them under control, which sometimes means ignoring some behaviors. For example, they may demand money unnecessarily to buy new fashions and designs to fit with their peers. If denied, they get angry and even refuse to eat or talk. In this situation, ignore their demands and provide what is necessary.

**b.** Teenagers tend to withdraw from their parents and associate with peers most. They are forming their identity and conviction about God, themselves, and life. Ensure you remain close and relevant so that you answer every question they may have to maintain your influence.

**c.** Teenagers tend to engage in risky behavior like substance use, unprotected sex, violence, unsafe recreational activities, peer influence, internet gaming, etc., because brains are not fully developed since parts responsible for judgment and decision-making are not fully mature. They, therefore, need guidance and control.

*Proverbs 11:14. where there is no counsel, the people fall, but in the multitude of counselors, there is safety*

**d.** Teenagers tend to lean on people who understand them, relate, and are relevant to their issues. They will often avoid judgmental people who pose to be perfect.

**e.** Teenagers tend to mind their personal space in terms of their rooms, clothes, fashion sense, time, hobbies, priorities, and decisions.

**f.** Teenagers are more concerned about their physical outlook, beauty, and fashion. They are in an era of fitting in with their peers and hence demand trending shoes, clothes, phones, and such.

**g.** In a healthy family setup, teenage boys tend to withdraw from their mother at an average age of 13 years to their father to be taught how to be a logical man. They watch how Dad treats Mum, values his work, and relates to them and others.

*Proverbs 4:20: My son attends to my words...*

Teenage girls tend to share and express their challenges, especially issues dealing with body image since they are emotional beings.

However, your relationship with them will depend on how attached you are during the previous stages of development. Some teenagers tend to withdraw entirely from their parents, who are too judgmental and never create a good relationship with them. When they withdraw, as a parent, draw closer to them and be part of their issues.

**Use the following tactics in parenting teenagers:**

**a. Be the Informer, personal coach, and director:** - Be the first to teach, mentor, and coach them to conform to the proper morals and standards. Start conversations on various topics like body changes, sexuality, healthy friendships, etc.

Let them understand the effects of associating with risky behavior like fornication, drug abuse, pornography, etc. Please keep the conversation open and assure them of your support whenever they face such issues. Our daughter, encountered a first hand with a lesbian who approached her to become her girlfriend. But since we had prepared her for it, and was well informed about it, she had the power to say no and even talked to the girl against it. She came and openly confided in us, and we were able to offer more guidance.

On the other hand, a girl confided in us about an issue she was going through. But she said her mother is so over-strict and unreasonable, and she can't confide in her. Why? Teenagers understand the language of friendship and mind much about being judged and condemned. Once you pose as a perfect parent, they tend to close and shift their concerns to peers or other people who understand them, and, in the process, many are taken advantage of or abused.

> *Teenagers understand the language of friendship*

b. **A balance between influence and control** - The level of influence comes when the teen is fully convinced that the parent understands and loves them, is non-judgmental, and means well to them. Therefore, even if you control them, they comply willingly at a level of love. The critical fact is that teenagers don't seek to be controlled fully or be left on their own to practice what they wish; all they desire is to be guided on the right path.

At this level, let them understand the dos and don'ts of the family. These are regulations from the family that no one is supposed to go against. For example, as a teenager, you are not supposed to impregnate or get pregnant at an early age. We stated earlier that many communities have taboos and code of conduct that regulates children from engaging in sex before marriage since they would be regarded as an outcast. This would go along way to curb today's menace of early teenage pregnancy. These cultural conducts were in line with scriptural guidelines. - **Exodus***22: 16.*

**c. Grant them freedom but set limits;** -Teenagers feel an increased need for privacy and liberty. They may start to explore ways of being independent through fashion choices, hobbies, and friends to engage with, which sometimes may be contrary to their parents. In this process, they may disregard boundaries and react strongly if parents or guardians reinforce limits. Give them the freedom to make their own decisions but, on the other hand, offer rules and boundaries that they should not go against. Teenagers crave for independence.

Let them know their limits concerning freedom of association, freedom of expression, freedom of choice, freedom of dressing etc. This gives them a sense of direction and limits external influences, which sometimes become problematic since they know what to do. **Be supportive and set clear limits with high (but reasonable) expectations.**

Communicate clearly and have reasonable expectations for school engagement, media use and behavior. At the same time, gradually expanding opportunities for more independence over time as your child takes on responsibility. Youth with parents who aim for this balance have been shown to have lower rates of depression and drug use.

## Stage 5

## Counselor and Friendship 18+ years.

This is the entry level of adulthood. I assume this child is out of secondary school and will probably proceed to college or university or join the work industry. The child here is mature enough to make their own decisions. There is no active parenting here since they are independent and on their own. Guide them, advise them, pray for them, and help them in making choices in their career, relationships, marriages, and investments.

There is a caution at this stage; many parents release their children into the world to concentrate on other siblings. These children are forced to independently move out and look for greener pastures and education. As they struggle to make their lives better, many have fallen victim to circumstances, abuse, manipulation, and bad choices which has led to many losing their star of destiny.

Therefore, at this age, support them especially financially. Make sure their lives are covered to create no room for intruders. Many children make mistakes at this level, especially when parents can't educate and cater to their needs. A 19-year-old studying at a local university said that her mother gives her enough money to cater for herself. Therefore, no man can come to confuse her with cash in exchange of her precious dignity.

Joshua in the bible is a practical example who was confident in his parenting, and he knew that they would serve the Lord together with his family. This is after leading the Israelites in **Joshua 24:14-15**, he said,

*"Fear the LORD and serve him with all faithfulness. Throw away the gods your ancestors worshiped beyond the Euphrates River and in Egypt, and serve the LORD. but if serving the LORD seems undesirable to you, choose for yourselves this day whom you will serve, whether the gods your ancestors served beyond the Euphrates or the gods of the Amorites, in whose land you are living. But as for me and my household, we will serve the lord."*

In conclusion, parenting has no end or graduation because you carry it on to your grandchildren. Therefore, successful parenting is when you see your grownup children strongly rooted in God, and they raise their children well. Also, you remain influential and instrumental to them even when living their separate lives. We often hear children confess that if it were not for my parents, my life could be a living hell. This shall become your portion in Jesus' mighty name.

# *Chapter 4*

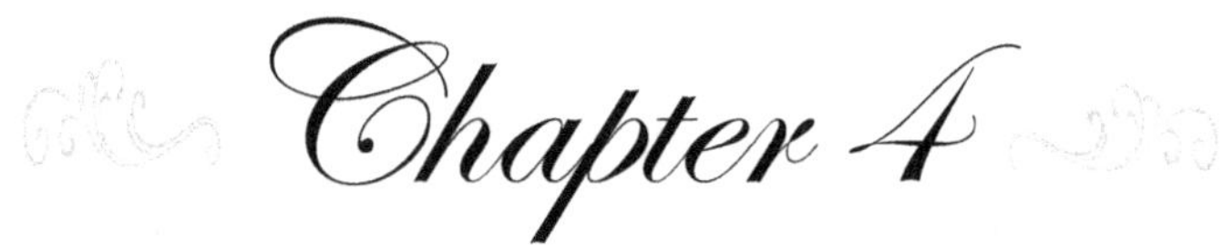

## Essential Gifts for Parental Inheritance

*Proverbs 13:22: A good man leaves an inheritance to his grandchildren.*

Inheritance refers to what one receives by succession as the heir (legal entitlement). This doesn't only refer to physical things but also in terms of properties, conditions, or a trait from the parent to the children. Education and career are important, but other hidden gifts can make your child excel higher to carry on your legacy. This can be done through training.

*Proverbs 22:6 Train up a child in the way he should go and once he grows up, he will not depart from it.*

Training means equipping or teaching a person a particular skill or behavior. A trained athlete will manifest in an event through results that require time, dedication, diligence, and sacrifice. Also, the trainer possesses more skills and expertise to impact the trainees. This means a parent as a trainer must make the children conform to their principles to remain the influencer. It is showing them the way to follow.

The quality of training in a child determines the quality of life they will live. Many children have missed many opportunities due to a lack of proper training from their parents. Other children will always avoid a misbehaving child. Other parents in the neighborhood will be cautioning their children against associating with them. Therefore, training is critical to ensuring children are equipped

> *The quality of training in a child determines the quality of life they will live.*

with good qualities and character that will enable them to fulfill their destiny quickly and add value to themselves, the kingdom of God, and our nation.

A man is a triune being, meaning he is composed of the spirit (spiritual), soul (emotions, feelings, and mind), and body (physical). All these aspects must be developed to ensure a balance in the child's development. Many parents have invested in physical things only, neglecting crucial elements that have raised an empty generation. Therefore, if you desire to raise children that will carry your legacy to generations, you must transfer the following gifts as inheritance.

## 1. Spiritual Mantles and Anointings.

God made man in His image *(Genesis 1:26)* and imparted his spirit in him. *In John 4: 24 - God is a Spirit: and they that worship him must worship him in spirit and truth.*

In order of priority, the spiritual part should be invested heavily to control every other aspect of a man. - *1Thessalonians 5;23.*

The most significant investment you can leave for your children is Jesus because He is all.  In our upbringing, we lacked many goodies, but our parents pushed us to church. That spiritual investment is what is speaking for us today. Spiritual mantles ensure that children enjoy the benefits of GOD, which money can't buy. This includes parental blessings **(Ephesians 6;1)**, Godly morals and character **(Galatians 5;22-23)**, Preserved destiny and purpose **(Jeremiah 29;11)**, Access to long life **(Deuteronomy 5;33, Ephesians 6;1-4)**, Access to favor **(Psalms 90;17. Psalms 5;12,**

**Psalms 84;11)**, Preserved generation. **Psalms 112:2-3, Genesis 17:7,** Access to health and wholeness.

**Jeremiah 30; 17.** This generation requires God. The devil is in the business of destroying them.

Therefore, equipping should begin from childhood. Let your children know Jesus early because that system will become part of them, bearing in mind that any untrained aspects will become difficult to follow. Many people struggle to pray before eating simply because that system was never introduced during childhood. A child has the mental capability to learn. If a child can operate a smartphone more than the parent at the age of five years, they can understand Jesus.

This is done through home evening devotions, Sunday school, and youth ministry. Begin by reading simple scriptures, explain to them based on their understanding, and let them recite simple bible verses, pray, and sing together. This system will start shaping their perspective in life by understanding that God is the source and author of everything. Spirituality regulates and dominates 100% of children's behavior.

**How do we invest spiritually?**

a. Lead them to have a personal relationship with Jesus(salvation) **Romans 10:9-10**. This should be done after careful explanation and understanding of the scripture. It is not to be imposed.

b.	Lead them to the baptism of the Spirit. **Acts 1:8.**

c.	Help them to develop a Christian character through the word of God. For example, honesty, diligence, and integrity. **Mark 7:23, Hebrews 4:12**

d.	Guide them to discover and understand God's will for their lives **Jeremiah 1:5.** Their mission and purpose. This can be done by finding their passion, talents, and inner strengths. Channel them in that direction. We see children becoming preachers and song ministers at an early age of 10 years.

e.	Help them find their place of service – getting involved in the house of God, Sunday school, teens department, sanctuary keepers, ushers. **Exodus 23:25** – a reward for their service is sure.

f.	Leading by example: Children are natural mimics. They hear what they observe more than what you teach. Let them see you are active in service; they will automatically develop a hunger for service.   **1 Timothy 4;12.**

g.	Sow a positive seed, and talk well of them. Let them know their identity in Christ. This will raise their confidence and esteem to work out their life. Jacob's pronouncement to Reuben in **Genesis 49;4** came to pass in **1 Chronicles 5;1)**

h.      Teach them spiritual weapons to destroy the works of the devil once enemies of their destiny challenge them: the blood of Jesus and the name of Jesus.

## 2. Personal Convictions.

This is the sum of your values, beliefs, philosophies, opinions, ideas, and mind systems. This is a personal creed, revelation, or faith regarding life.  Every parent in every family possesses these traits, which shape their destinies and way of life.

In **Genesis 18:17-19** God knew that Abraham would transfer spiritual convictions to his children.

Personal convictions are molded by our daily walks and investment in ourselves spiritually. To be like Jesus, you must know his walks and traits.

*In Deuteronomy 6; 1, 2, 7, 20 and 21.* God gave the Israelites the commandments (verse 1) and commanded them to teach their children (verse 7), which served as generational convictions (verses 20 & 21).

As a parent, what do you believe about God, Satan, failure, success, excellence, wealth, poverty, challenges, and victory? It should be replicated in your children. These philosophies will form your convictions. This explains why children of politicians, pastors, and businesspeople become like their parents. Transfer business convictions, spiritual and political convictions, good values, and the success you desire your children to possess. This will help them choose their paths right.

This also implies negative convictions. ***Proverbs 23:7 As he thinketh in his heart, so is he:***

Today, we see very wealthy and great families' empires collapsing once their parents die. This happens because they didn't prepare or equip them well with skills to run these empires.  Let them learn through your journey of success and challenges. This will impact a success mindset and a fighting spirit to handle challenges.  We are blessed once we see Bishop David Oyedepo's (founder of Living Faith International) children preaching the gospel powerfully. This never comes through impartation only but through training and daily walk with God.

**Luke 15:11-32** narrates a story of the prodigal son who squandered all his inheritance. He had physical things but not

> *Any successful man is a product of their positive convictions*

business convictions that could have helped him to make more wealth. As a parent, never retire without transferring Godly and positive convictions to your children.

**Important Note:** *Any successful man is the product of their positive convictions.*

## 3. Good Name.

A name carries your impact, track record, contribution, and credibility. A name is like a **price tag** for identity. Names are **keys** to unlock doors of success and opportunities. Today, once you visit a supermarket, we often look for certain brands of products simply because we are convinced, they are of good quality.

 God concentrated on making Abraham a generational blessing through his name. *Genesis 12:2 I will make you into a great nation, and I will bless you, I will make your name great, and you will be a blessing,*

**Names carry power and authority**. Jesus gave us His name so we can access any door we desire. *John 14:13-14, John 16:23-24, Mark 16:17, Acts 3:6.*

This is true even here on earth since there are names you can mention, and you get a job, scholarship, opportunity, tender, or business favor directly. We have enjoyed this favor where GOD has elevated us to the point of rubbing shoulders with kings and great people in our Republic. Therefore, as a parent, a good name will pave the way for your generation.

**Proverbs** *22:1. A good name is more desirable than great riches; to be esteemed is better than silver or gold.*

We have witnessed children enjoying favor from the community after the death of their parents since they were so charitable to people in the estate. A good name is wealth; our children have enjoyed favor due to our good deeds. Names are generational investments and can be used as a point of reference.

*Ecclesiastes 7:1 A good name is better than fine perfume.*

We have enjoyed blessings due to our parents charitable works, which they passed onto us

On the other hand, a bad name can be padlocked to lock destinies and multiply hardships and pain. Some parents have ruined their children's destinies due to bad names.

Therefore, the best gift you can give your children is your good name by living well with people, helping them, respecting and honoring them. Look around your surroundings and see the children of that womanizer, killer, rude, disrespectful, stingy, and conflictual family.  One time, We had a fierce neighbor who was always rude and disrespectful to the neighbors. Children in the vicinity would play, celebrate birthdays together, and exclude her children.

> *Names Speak Even in Death.*

Our prayer is that your name will be a key in Jesus name.

*Important Note: Names Speak Even in Death.*

## 4. Inner Beauty.

This is the invisible aspect of a man but is physically reflected through actions or behavior.

*Luke 6:45 A good man brings good things out of the good stored up in his heart, and an evil man brings evil things out of the evil stored up in his heart. For the mouth speaks what the heart is full of".*

In parenting, grow this aspect in your children by ensuring they are impressive inside and out. Don't just feed your children and clothe them with expensive designer clothes; let their inner beauty be reflected outwardly.

Have you encountered a very handsome, learned and wealthy man wearing expensive clothes but with an evil heart. These people are alienated, and everybody runs away from them because they possess a very toxic personality. That's why the bible cautions us against looking at physical beauty. **Proverbs** *31:30 beauty can be deceptive.*

God is more interested in our inner man, which should be prioritized.

*1 Samuel 16:7 But the LORD said to Samuel, "Do not consider his appearance or his height, for I have rejected him. The LORD does not look at the things people look at. People look at the outward appearance, but the LORD looks at the heart."*

The apostle Peter admonished Christians not to focus only on physical beauty but also inwardly.**1 Peter 3:3-4.** This has denied many people God's blessings and favor from men due to their inner filthiness. Everyone wants to stay close to a jovial, goodhearted, kind, organized, and respectful person. They sent a sweet fragrance into the air.

**Inner beauty is seen in the following areas:**

1.      Modesty dressing, not seductively. This has become an issue, especially in the modern generation, where they dress, exposing all their private parts, not even considering whether they are grown-ups in their midst, including in the house of God.

*Proverbs. 7:10 –and behold they met him a woman with the attire of a harlot and subtle of heart.*

2.      Good in academics and delivering results. Also, they understand their career paths well based on their passion and talents.

3.      They portray a good home environment by maintaining cleanliness, order, and neatness in their rooms and bodies. Let them learn how to cook and do house chores even in places where there is house help.

4.      They have inner joy, peace, and happiness, which shows they are free from pain and trauma. **Nehemiah 8:10, Isaiah 41:10, proverbs 17:22**

5.      Good managers of time, resources, and themselves. This is by having a schedule per day.  A balanced day should have wake-up time, homework time, eating time, revision time, playing time, relaxing time, house chores time, and watching time.

6.      A good character in terms of respect, humility, and obedience.

7.      **Emotional Stability and Intelligence.**

This aspect is found in a man's soul. It's an aspect that helps people express their feelings and control their emotions towards themselves and others. Children whose emotions are nurtured positively develop trust, self-control, and a positive attitude.

**Let's discuss shortly how you develop your children's emotional stability.**

**1.      Develop mechanisms to control anger, resentment, and bitterness**: Teach your children to act reasonably without being offended when provoked. When they exhibit resentment and tantrums, help them tame themselves over time, they will be stable. This explains why many people have lost opportunities, valuable relationships, friendships, connections, and jobs due to a lack of emotional control. The root cause of anger and bitterness emanates from childhood pressures and trauma. Anger is the incubation of unresolved issues like trauma, family conflicts, lack of love, and rejection. - *Ephesians 4:26-32:*

Many children are suffering due to their parent's unresolved anger, which is projected toward them. Also, if the father and mother have marital conflicts, children suffer the most. One teenage girl confessed to us that she had a mission to kill her angry father because he used to beat her mother, which led to health complications until she passed on.

Secondly, we encountered a lady who suffered a nasty breakup from a previous relationship. She projected the anger to her child since her presence could remind her of the man who betrayed her. She used to discipline her child ruthlessly, even sometimes without any reason. One day, as she was beating her, she hit her against the wall, and the baby died. She is now serving jail due to murder charges in Prison. Just imagine if that child survived and was brought up in that toxic environment. She could have grown to be an angry, rejected, and bitter girl who would release the same negative energy to others.

Therefore, if you desire to raise emotionally stable children, begin by practicing the act of forgiveness and letting go of any wrongs done against you. - *Mark 11:25*

Purpose to release every person who wronged you, that father who rejected you after birth, that man who raped you, that wife or husband who took advantage of you in marriage. This is because children develop control by just watching how you handle them and the people around you. Anger leads to evil and destruction. *Psalms 37:8*

*Ephesians 6:4And, ye fathers, provoke not your children to wrath: but bring them up in the nurture and admonition of the Lord.*

**2.     Teach them how to control their sexual emotions, especially teenagers,** by keeping Christian friends and shunning intimate relationships. Teach them the act of saying NO to sexual gestures.

*2 Timothy 2:22 flee also youthful lust, but follow righteousness, faith, charity, peace, with them that call on the lord out of pure heart.*

This is probably the leading cause of sexual immorality proliferation in this modern generation. Many young people are messing up their lives due to a lack of emotional intelligence. Admonish them never to give their mind a break but always think straight and reasonably when encountering such situations. This calls for sex talk with your children.

**3.     Please help them to develop openness by expressing their emotions because it's normal.**

Sometimes, they may be happy, angry, bored, bitter, or confused. Please help them to handle these emotions to strike a balance. Especially for teenagers who experience a range of emotions tend to get angry once they need something. Once challenged, others resolve to cut themselves in their arms and thighs, run away from home, they get silent and withdraw from everyone to get your attention.  This is an unhealthy way of expressing their emotions. Admonish them to talk and highlight their issues once they cool down so they can be helped.

**4.      Model to them how to empathize and understand themselves and others.** This is being human and merciful by treating others with love and humanity. People who develop this unsympathetic disorder show low emotional intelligence and stress within themselves. They fail to grasp that the person they hurt doesn't contribute to their pain; they are happy when they hurt others.

Good emotional development will bring balance to your children as they become mature, reasonable, and controllable beings who can make intelligent decisions.
- **Proverbs 14:29**

i.                    **Good Character.**

This refers to cultivating and building unique traits and characteristics in a child. Character is what defines a person. Talent and qualifications

> *Good Character is their first paycheck; it will open doors of success and favor.*

can take you to the top, but character keeps you there. These traits include respect, accountability, responsibility, authority, hard work, honesty, and integrity.

*Proverbs 12:22 Lying lips are an abomination to the LORD: but they that deal truly are his delight.*

Good character is their first paycheck; it will open doors of success and favor in their lives.

*Proverbs 10:9 He that walketh uprightly walketh surely: but he that perverteth his ways shall be known."*

How many people have lost opportunities and favors due to a lack of honesty and integrity?

This is the reason behind many social problems we are experiencing in our country. Such as corruption, sexual perversion, immorality, irresponsibility, and deviance. Good character will preserve your children's destinies.

*Proverbs 11:3The integrity of the upright shall guide them: but the perverseness of transgressors shall destroy them.*

**How do you build character?**

a.      **Watch your character as a parent**. Children aspire to be like you. They watch every character you exhibit to them and others, too. If you are ruthless towards people, they will emulate you. How can you advise your son against drugs and alcohol when you are a drunkard? How can you guide and direct marriage while you are fighting daily? Parenting is by influence and modeling. Please do what you want them to learn, and consciously, they follow.

*Philippians 4:8-9* advises believers to focus on things that are true, honest, just, pure, lovely, and of good report. They should also contemplate virtues and praise-worthy matters. Additionally, the passage encourages adherents to follow the examples set by the speaker, with the promise that the God of peace will be with them.

**1 Corinthians 15:33 states that character is learned.** *Be not deceived: evil communications corrupt good manners."*

## b. Build a family culture.

Family culture states a defined or specific way or methodology of doing things within the family.  For example, a praying culture is cultivated through having fellowships and praying before eating or sleeping.  If you desire your children to have integrity, teach them honesty and transparency. Family culture entails having a culture of responsibility, time, respect, performance, honesty, transparency, and discipline. With clear goals and purpose, this system becomes part of their lives.

Once we visited a home in the village, and when food was served, the child began picking meat from visitor plates. What surprised us, the mother just watched, and supported the act, justifying that the son loves meat. We were so pissed off, but we couldn't alter a word. But what lingered in our minds was whether this child was ever taught how to handle visitors. Children can shame you if you don't teach them manners, especially in the presence of other people. They can talk about anything and everything, including secrets.

We see how Joseph in *Genesis 39:9* exhibited sexual ethics, honor, and respect towards his master's wife, who had intended to trap him in sexual sin. He would have lost his glorious destiny. We also see Daniel, who exhibited spiritual discipline when he purposed to remain on the side of God and refused to compromise.

*Daniel 1:8* states that Daniel resolved in his heart not to eat the king's food or drink his wine, so he asked the chief official for permission to avoid defiling himself in this manner. God used and preserved his destiny.

### c. Maintain consistency when teaching behavior.
Keep on doing it over time. Correct the behavior all the time so that they can grasp the methodology. It is crucial to maintain balance in your parenting. If the father says no to any demand, it should be the same for the mother. This closes the element of comparison between the children.

*Galatians 6:9 and let us not be weary in well doing, for in due season we shall reap if we faint not.*

## d. Goal setting and monitoring

Have targets for your children based on the character you desire them to possess. For example, to pass their exams, lead them through revision and extra tuition, and make sure you monitor everything. Once they perform, this will condition them to believe in the value of hard work, excellence, and goal setting. Once they achieve, appreciate and sometimes reward their hard work. It encourages the outcome of the same behavior.

*Habakkuk 2:2 and the lord answered me and said, write a vision and make it plain upon tables that he may run that readeth it."*

One married woman in the church said that she finds it an abomination to return to her house past 7 pm because it was a rule in their father's house that no one could return after 6 pm unless under permission for unavoidable reasons. This has helped her till now. Therefore, set the standards of character that you desire your children to possess. It will help them big time.

## e. **Set boundaries and administer discipline when deviated**

This involves correcting with love without manipulation or abuse.

*Proverbs 13:24. he who spares his rod hates his son.*

Sometimes, overlook their behavior and encourage them to do the right thing. And once they attain your desired trait, reward them to encourage more positive behavior. Be aware of abuse, whether physical or verbal. Correction should be done with love and warmth. This will ensure that you live in peace and harmony.

*Proverbs 29:15 The rod of correction imparts wisdom, but a child left to himself disgraces his mother. Verse 17: discipline your son, and he will give you peace and delight to your soul.*

j.      **Mental Horsepower.**

Increasing mental horsepower entails enlarging their cognitive capacity. Human beings possess mental faculties that help them reason, be creative, think logically, imagine, and shape their perceptions and attitudes. Whatever information the brain absorbs, either by sight or hearing, forms the thought systems reflected in our physical lives. Therefore, your thought system's quality equals your life's quality.

*Proverbs 23:7 For as he thinketh in his heart, so is he.*

The mind is a memory tank. It is the battlefield of everything in life. The information absorbed, whether audio or visual, is stored in the subconscious mind, which, when repeatedly practiced, becomes your belief system and life patterns. Belief systems define us and drive our decisions and behavior.

*Mathew 12:34 For out of the abundance of the heart the mouth speaketh.*

Whatever proceeds in your mouth is what is in your thought system. Information is the food of the brain, which shapes their mindset—every child with an inferior or failing mindset results from the influence of the surroundings. The mind is the only organ traveling into your future; it's the control valve. Therefore, every dream and aspiration must be seen and born in the mind.

Today, the influence of social media and digitalization has played a significant role in shaping the mindset of our children. They want to be like people they see in cartoons. My second-born daughter watches her favorite cartoon, Diana and Roma.  This has changed her to the point she wants to dress like her, do make-up like her, and make her room resemble hers. In short, she wants to be Diana. Children are living in a world of fantasy.

It is important to note that the capacity for thinking has been reduced and conditioned to the level of social media. This has resulted in mentally weak children with no ideas and creativity. We have seen a mentally handicapped generation in which even making a simple decision is a problem. This is evident due to the high rate of unemployment in a society where more than 20 million graduates are jobless. This shows that the rate of creativity is low since everybody wants to be employed rather than create opportunities. Poverty and success are a product of the mind.

That's why you can give a mentally poor person one million shillings/dollars, and after a short time, the person goes back to the same state. A student can get an A in a village school with no resources. This is the product of the mind.

Additionally, the rate of suicide among young people due to mental illnesses shows a low level of mental toughness, which helps people deal with pressures, stress, and challenges regardless of the circumstances. The rate of anti-social behavior shows negative influences and poor mindsets.

Mentally strong children are high achievers; they are disciplined and possess a high sense of value, direction, vision, and mindset. They have a positive attitude towards themselves and life. Hence, they are less likely to be mentally ill or involved in anti-social behavior since they know their identity and values well. Today, we live in a highly intellectual world where scammers eat out of other people's foolishness. This is vital to ensure your kid survives in this tactful world. It is important, whenever possible, to take your children to schools that have programs that increase your children's mental exposure.

How can you build a mentally strong generation with the right mindset?

a.      **Help your children view life through the lens of the word of God**. Let them know their self-identity, worth, and aspirations based on the word of God. Let them know the purpose and reason of their creation.
Let them answer these questions; -

Who am I? (identity)
Why am I here? (purpose)
Where am I from? (source)
Where am I going? (Destiny)

This will help them discover their true identity, source, purpose, and destination.

*Hosea 2:6My people are destroyed for lack of knowledge: because thou hast rejected knowledge.*

This knowledge will shape their mentality to strive and be the best.

**b.** **Regulate the kind of information they absorb** from the mass and social media. Whatever you feed your mind empowers your thinking and becomes your life.

*Proverbs 23:7For as he thinketh in his heart, so is he:* The quality of your life reflects the quality of your thoughts. When thoughts are repeated, they make one a master in a specific behavior. For example, mastering driving or swimming needs consistency, patience, and more practice. Therefore, if they feed their mind with wrong information automatically, their behavior will correspond with their wrong thinking patterns, and their actions will be failure and frustration. You can't think of failure and success.

**c.** **Exposure**–exposure brings hidden things to the surface and allows one to see the world from a broader perspective.  It helps us see more new opportunities and challenge our realities. It stirs our minds to move out of our comfort zone. Expose them to places that will trigger their mental capacity to enlarge their brain capacity.

A child with a defeatist mentality can possess a positive mentality by associating with right-minded people and feeding on positive information.  Expose them to programs and places that will trigger their mental capacity.  This creates their curiosity and motivation to work hard and achieve more.

**d.     Help them reframe their thoughts** when they face a challenge. This involves thinking realistically and interpreting a situation from different perspectives, especially encouraging them always to think positively. This may include helping them remove wrong mindsets like negative attitudes and failure mindsets.

It also involves eliminating thoughts against themselves and transforming their minds.

*Romans 12:2 and be not conformed to this world but be ye transformed by the renewing of your mind, that ye may prove what is that good and acceptable and perfect will of God.*

**e.     Build their mental muscles** by creating an innovative and creative attitude in them. This involves thinking outside the box.  This is done by assigning more tasks, setting deadlines, and probably tasks higher than them. This will trigger their thinking capacity, force them to think beyond the norm when they cannot, and assist them by breaking the task into smaller achievable tasks. This can be done by reading story books, watching educational documentaries, and participating in contests like spelling bees and trivia.

**f.     Empower their imagination**. Imagination is a faculty in the mind that forms new ideas and images of things not present now. This entails drawing their future in their mind.

*Genesis 11:6- And the L*ORD *said, Behold, the people is one, and they have all one language; and this they begin to do: and now nothing will be restrained from them, which they have imagined to do.*

This scripture highlights a story of people building the tower of Babel. The Lord said that nothing they imagined would be refrained from them. So, whatever is too big for your imagination is too big for your destination. It begins from your mind. Please help them to see themselves bigger and greater.

k.      **Association** -Encourage them to associate with friends and peers with a positive mindset. Please encourage them to have role models, mentors, and people who will help them become achievers in life.

*Proverbs 27:17 As iron sharpens iron, so one person sharpens another.*

l.      **Your Relationships and Social Connections.**

Associations with peers and adults affect how children think, learn, and develop. Families, schools, and peer groups all make up an essential part of their social context. We are social beings and can't live without one another. Help your children cultivate positive **social capital** within themselves, their peers, relatives, teachers, and the community. Please help them to choose friends and understand the need for positive peer influence. Positive peer influence molds positive behavior and helps in making intelligent choices. **Proverbs 13:20, proverbs 27;17.**

Please help them know the value of social capital and how to live well with and respect them. I have seen situations where friends have become destiny helpers.

**Genesis 12:1** - Abraham was a destiny helper to his cousin Lot.  Earlier in our school, We witnessed a parent paying school fees for their daughter's best friend, who was financially challenged.

As a parent, connect your children to families within your social circle. As these children interact, they create a social class connection to help them.  We can travel far to attend a birthday party for a 1-year-old baby of our friend with our children to help them connect with other children.  Your connection is your net worth.

Establish guardrails and cautions, shield them against negative peer influence, which sways people towards risky activities like criminal behaviors, drug abuse, and other unhealthy lifestyles.

*1 Corinthians 15:33 – do not be deceived; bad company corrupts good character.*

We have handled cases of drug abuse, lesbianism, masturbation, and pornography addiction. Among young people to whom their peers introduced them.

**2 Kings 12:10** highlights the story of Rehoboam, who was misled by his friends and ended up losing his throne.

m.      **Security and Stability.**

Every human being needs to feel safe and away from harm. This entails making sure that your children are free and secure from threats.  We are living in a dangerous society where insecurity is on the rise. It isn't easy to trust anyone with your children. I have handled many cases of child abuse emanating from parents, relatives, house managers, and neighbors.

As parents, be sure of whoever you are leaving your children with.  **Samuel 19:11- 12** – highlights the story of a mother named Michal, warning his son, David, of assassins who plan to eliminate him. In Genesis **21:9-12, Ishmael mocked Isaac,** but Sarah defended him.  Prayerfully, confront every assassin and Ishmael mocking the destiny of your children, which may be negative peer pressure, wrong mindsets, lesbianism, fornication, drugs, or gambling.

Additionally, learn to listen to your children and be vigilant to notice any change in them.  In our career, out of ten cases of depression we handle, seven cases emanate from sexual violence. One girl confessed that her biological dad began abusing her sexually at the early age of 10 years. And the moment she told the mother, she didn't believe her. The mother hated her and could punish her ruthlessly to the point she broke a bone in her body. We met this girl three years ago when she was plotting to commit suicide because of depression. The doctor confirmed that she can't bear children due to four abortions she carried out earlier. She is HIV positive and is now living somewhere without a family, and recently, she was confirmed to have breast cancer. She was so bitter to the verge of planning to kill her dad.

Another boy opened up that his Choir master assaulted him sexually, but he fears confiding to his parents since the abuser is a family friend.  The question is, what do you think the future holds for these children? The trauma they have faced will affect their lives negatively for good.

**I give the following recommendations to assist you as a parent in securing your children.**

1.      Educate them on our dangerous times and caution them against anybody who may try to harm them: strangers, relatives, house managers, etc.

2.      Limit their movements. Let them stay in their homes or play outside under surveillance. Why do you let children

go to other people's houses in the village alone and leave them with relatives you don't have a track record of their character and life? This exposes your children to the risk of abuse physically, sexually, or emotionally.

3.      Admonish them against talking to strangers or receiving gifts from them because they use drugs to intoxicate them and lure them into sexual assault.

4.      Teach them the worth of their body parts. And no one should see and touch them since it's a holy temple of God. - *1Corinthians 3:16*

5.      Also, dress them appropriately by covering their body. Also, teach them to sit nicely to avoid provoking assault against themselves. - *Proverbs 7:10*

6.      Also, they should shout or seek help if they face such compromising situations. This is because abusers threaten to kill them once they are exposed. Let them know there is help.

7.      Above all, pray for your children daily before they leave for school and cover them with the blood of Jesus. No devil can touch an anointed child.

*Galatians 6:17 From henceforth let no man trouble me: for I bear in my body the marks of the Lord Jesus.*

n.      **<u>Love and belonging.</u>**

Every child has a need to be loved, appreciated, and accepted. Love makes children grow healthier, increases brain development, raises their esteem, and improves their grades.  This is done by cultivating warmth early by showing affection, having mutual activities, and offering support when needed. This creates strong bonds between parents and children, which will help them become less fearful of the world around them.

Children raised in cold homes where fathers are dictators and mothers are disciplinarians develop an Inferiority complex, which is a psychological deficiency. They often feel unloved and insecure, have low self-worth, and always seek validation and approval from everyone.  As a result, these children develop personality disorders and mental illnesses, which make them live an unfulfilled life.

Today, we live in a generation that values how their parents make them feel (emotional aspect) rather than logically thinking about the sacrifice you make for them. A child today can feel unloved simply because his brother has more shoes than him. Additionally, if you correct them, they interpret them as being unloved.  This is where we strike a balance: treat your children in a manner that will not make them feel less.

## How to cultivate love in your children:

1.      Let them know the unconditional love of God towards them. *John 3;16, Isaiah 54;10 and Romans 5:8*

2.      Tell them that you love them, appreciate them, reward them, and acknowledge their little achievements.

3.      Love one another as parents; children are imitators.

4.      Don't compare your children with anyone else. Instead, appreciate their uniqueness and help them overcome their weaknesses with love.

5.      Cease yelling at them at all times.

6.      Please don't call them names, as this negatively affects their mindset. Your words are like arrows. They can destroy or build your children.

Many children who grow up with a love deficit always seek approval from their friends. These children will always have a vacuum if the love void is not filled. They tend to do too much to prove themselves worthy and maintain friendships including the wrong ones.

For example, girls raised by single mothers who have love deficits tend to date older men since they are looking for a father's love, which they never had. In short, they are vulnerable to abuse. Imagine this scenario: If Jesus died for our sins because of love for humanity, and if two different people can be joined in marriage due to love, that's how love is magical and robust.

**Songs of Songs 8:6b Love is as strong as death.**

Please give it to them unconditionally, even when they are going astray. Love can change a negative behavior.

o. **Identity.**

*Identity is a price tag. It's the only thing that brings true happiness.*

Identity is knowing who we are, our goals, passions, and aspirations. It entails the uniqueness of a person. Identity defines us and our dreams in life. It helps us view ourselves from the maker's perspective because God created us uniquely and purposefully. Help

> *Identity is a price tag; It's the only thing that brings true happiness.*

your children to view themselves through their manufacturer (God) manual(bible).

Today, young people have **identity crises** due to peer and internet influence. Every youth has a famous person they want to imitate. This has brought so much chaos, and the devil is using this to pass his evil agenda in the world. Look at the issues of Lesbians and gays. How can two men and women claim to form a family? They are going to the extent of questioning their natural body makeup. This is ridiculous. This is what identity crisis entails; it brainwashes.

If your children don't know who they are, the devil and the world will teach them who they are not. Identity helps your children to know who they are, build motivation towards achieving their goals and aspirations, and breed confidence to face life. Every negative behavior shows a lack of self-identity.

*Hosea 4:6* conveys that the people are suffering because they lack knowledge. This is because they have rejected knowledge, so they will be rejected as priests. Since they have forgotten God's law, He will also forget their children.

**How to build self-identity in children.**

1.    Teach them about their **Body image.** To appreciate their physical outlook since God made them just like they are.

*Psalms 139:13-14. I will praise thee; for I am fearfully and wonderfully made: marvelous are thy works; and that my soul knoweth right well.*

This awareness translates into confidence in them. The reason why people are paying millions of money to change their body makeup through surgery is a lack of self-love and who they are.

**2. Help them raise their Self-esteem** – to have confidence in themselves and God that there is nothing they can't achieve.

*Philippians 4:13, I can do all things through Christ which strengthens me. Hebrews 10:35-36.*

3. **Help them improve their self-image; this** is how they see themselves. If children feel loved, they will act and give love; if they see themselves as achievers, they can conquer to achieve. The parent's upbringing shapes this. Please help them see the good in themselves even when the situation proves otherwise. **Philippians 4-6:7**, the bible admonishes us not to be anxious about anything, but through prayer and supplication, every request be known to God, and He fulfills.

4. **Self-aspirations** – refer to their dreams and passions in life. Assure them of their glorious destiny in Christ. **Joshua 1:9.** Help them to build their names and careers to the point of actualization. This brings stability, confidence, and success in their lives. Identity is the first paycheck of

every child. Knowing who they are will make them conquer the world.

## 12.    Physical Assets.

Physical assets are tangible or material possessions like money, land, a house, a car, and a business. This will help them to have a startup. *Proverbs 13:22a* states that *A good man leaveth an inheritance to his children's children:* we see Abraham giving his physical inheritance to his children.

*Genesis25:5- 6: And Abraham gave all that he had unto Isaac. But unto the sons of the concubines, which Abraham had, Abraham gave gifts, and sent them away from Isaac his son, while he yet lived, eastward, unto the east country.*

This will assist them to have a foundation in their lives. We have seen children who have inherited their parents' companies and businesses, which saves them from long hassle. We desire to be the last people to be employed in our generation, which pushes us to work hard and create an empire for our children, who will pass it on to their children.

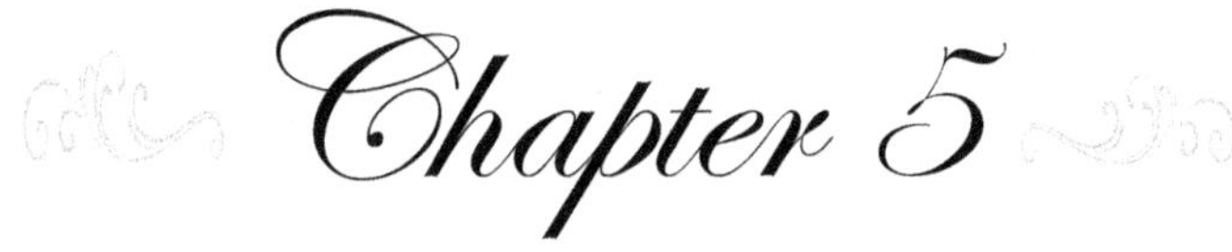

## Chapter 5

## Why God Desired Parenting to Be a Dual

Human being can reproduce just like animals and plants. But being good and responsible parents is what counts. The kind of parent you are will influence their life and inspire them to parent in the future.

Parenting is beyond provision. It's a full-time job with no vocational off, no retirement, no break; it's a continuous business. From the beginning, God intends for a child to be raised in a balanced home with both mother and father since each was given a specific assignment to instill in a child to raise Godly offspring *Malachi 2:15*. Children are products of marriage right from creation.

Today, the case is reversed. It's an era where children are raised in a valley of family crises. This includes those raised by single parents (father or mother); blended families where one is the biological parent; others by relatives like grandmother, aunties, and uncles; others abandoned in children's homes and streets; and co-parenting where parents are in their separate ways. And to make matters worse, the majority of those with both parents are raised under marital crisis. This has created gaps in these children's lives mentally and emotionally, breeding a very deviant bitter generation, boy child crisis, teenage pregnancies, drug addiction, crimes, rape, suicides, increase in mental health issues in children. But the truth is a child raised in a family of two serious, born-again, intentional parents and subjected to biblical principles becomes very successful and ends up having a great family.

Let us analyze the role of fathers and mothers in parenting from the mind of God;

## Fathers
**Father means Abba – which means source.** Fathers are the source of everything. In an organization, they are the Chief Executive Officers. They are the head. They give all to

children, from security, basic needs, guidance, direction, and assurance. Fathers model children how to run their families in the future.

The father teaches boys the value of becoming real men. This means taking on all the family responsibilities or caring for the wife and children. For girls, on the other hand, the father reflects the first man they will date or desire to be married to. They observe how daddy treats mummy.

Our first-born daughter desires to be married to a man like my husband since she sees a good man in him. That's why fathers are the first men to take their daughters for dates treat them and spend on them, especially and teach them how to handle a man in a relationship.

Especially today where girls are lured to friends-with-benefits relationships, especially when in college, used sexually, and become temporary wives where they cook, wash, and provide for men at a tender age. Finally, they are thrown out, frustrated, and broken. By then, you are the only safe and genuine man who can't harm your daughter. (Paragraph interchanged)

Fathers are the number one cheer leader, and their words of affirmation give children confidence three times that of their mothers. You can now imagine parenting without a father? Among many roles, this is what these children miss.

Many people admit that they struggled with feelings of abandonment and lack of direction, which made them turn to risky behavior like drugs, sex, and unhealthy relationships to numb the pain of fatherlessness.

This means that single mothers should strive to play both roles by delegating the role of a father to other male figures like grandfathers, uncles, cousins, and spiritual fathers. But this figure should be of good character to emulate and have good intentions.

Other roles of fathers in parenting include;

1.      **Spiritual priests** – they offer spiritual nourishment as the head of the family, just like Christ is the head of the church *Ephesians 5: 23.*

2.      **Identity** – Every generation is traced from the father's name—the generation of Joseph, Abraham. Fathers give children a sense of IDENTITY and ancestral roots. *John 16; 27-28.* Today, many identity certificates carry the mother's surname, an indication of absentee fathers in the family, which was not the will of God.

3.      **source of blessings and curses**:
God has entrusted fathers with the mandate to bless their children. In **Genesis 49:1-28,** we see Jacob blessing his 12 sons, whereas others were cursed due to disobedience. In

Verse 22, Joseph was blessed. A father figure blesses. That's why culture permits uncles or grandfathers to take that initiative in cases of absent fathers during occasions like weddings, initiation, and dowry.

In the case of curses, if children disobey the father, they automatically get a curse from God. **Genesis *49:3*** Reuben, the firstborn born, was cursed for defiling his father's bed. We have encountered a family who ganged against their father, amounting to nothing due to a curse. They toil day and night but have nothing to show for it.

Parents, be advised to keep your children away from your fights with their father because it can evoke curses towards them. In some cases, mothers always contribute this menace; kindly get wisdom and train your children to provoke blessings from their fathers.

### 4.      Gives leadership and direction.

From creation and culture, the father tops, then the wife and children complete the family. **In Genesis 2:24 - *Therefore shall a man leave his father and his mother and cleave unto his wife: and they shall be one flesh.*** Fathers are the leaders and carry the family's visions and dreams. They led the family to build a house, invest in health insurance, and educate the children.

A particular single lady has built a house worth 50 million. After sitting under a male mentor, she realized it was a solid, misplaced investment since she does not live there and works far away. The mentor advised her to set up businesses, which she has undertaken with great vigor.  She confesses that a lady without a husband is prone to make many mistakes. Single mothers are getting this wisdom and succeeding in raising very successful children.

Children learn about responsibility from their fathers. That's where boys are groomed to be real men.

## 5.	They Offer Security and Protection.

FATHERS offer security to the family. They shield the family from threats, hurt, pain, and financial constraints. Children feel safe when daddy is around. Our daughter always comes to report everyone who made fun of her in school to the dad.  She always says Daddy is so strong, which makes her feel secure. Children need to feel protected like an egg yolk in a shell... this gives them the confidence to face life because they have a shield by their side. This raises their self-esteem. A home with a father is respected and regarded with utmost regard, even in society.

## 6.	They Are Symbols of Authority and Commands.

Fathers are commanders in their homes. They give children a sense of authority in their lives. Men are naturally tough, and this instills resilience and a fighting virtue in children to enable them to face challenges with strength and vigor in the future. An example is Abraham, who was entrusted with a generation because God knew that he would command his children to keep the ways of the Lord. *Genesis 18:19*

We are living in callous and dangerous times. For children to make it in life, they need confidence, to be fearless, to know what they want to achieve, and to have the zeal to conquer the world without fear.

*2 Timothy 1:7 God has not given us the spirit of fear but of power and love and of sound mind.*

This virtue is trained and intentionally cultivated.

## 7.      Offer Instructions and Guidance

A father instructs and directs which way to be taken within the family. Children love to grow under a particular code of instructions that will make them actualize their destiny.

In **Genesis 50:16,** Jacob instructed Joseph to forgive his brothers before he died, and he obeyed. In Proverbs **1:8,** Father instructs. Genesis **24:34- 37**- Abraham had instructed a servant not to get a Canaanite wife for Isaac. Similarly, the bible cautions fathers against provoking their children in **Ephesians 6:4**but to instruct them in the Lord's ways.

## 8.      They offer discipline and correction.

Fathers correct and instill discipline in their children, guiding them on the right behaviors.

**1 Thessalonians 2:11-12** (*For you know that we dealt with each of you as a father deal with his own children, encouraging, comforting and urging(warning) you to live lives worthy of God, who calls you into his kingdom and glory.*

*Proverbs3:11-12. Proverbs 29:17;* Correct *thy son, and he shall give the rest; yea, he shall give delight unto thy soul.*

Mothers are naturally soft and nurturing; sometimes, instilling discipline in them is difficult. Fathers are strict and streamline children's behavior, especially boys, who sometimes grow to disrespect their mothers. Our daughter said that my mum is very soft but Daddy is tough, that's why she sometimes takes her phone without permission. Nobody forgets the disciplinary measures given by their father in their childhood.

## MOTHERS.

Mothers are so connected to children and nurturing, strengthening the bond naturally. Mothers biblically are mandated to raise children alongside the father as helpers.

But today, we are living in an era of absentee fathers, violent homes, and divorces where children are left under the care of their mothers to offer all their needs, creating a lot of parental gaps. Mothers have so many roles, but let highlight the crucial ones in the lives of children.

1. **Helper** – just like the Holy Spirit, mothers are helpers. They submit under the father's authority by ensuring every instruction given is followed to accomplishment. They help the father raise children by undertaking home duties such as cooking and cleaning. No one can forget their motherly training.

2. **Nurtures** –mothers naturally love and possess a strong connection with their children. They are the soft spot. Every child deeply connects with the mother which stabilizes their emotional needs. The connection speaks volumes.

3. **Teachers** – Mother teaches, **Proverbs 1:8.** They counsel and instill Godly values, order, cleanliness, personal grooming, and home chores.

4. **Prayer warrior** – She helps maintain a Godly atmosphere at home and a discerning spirit to know what's happening around the children. Alongside the husband ensures that church devotional programs are held at home. This will destroy all the strongholds of the devil to ensure

their destiny is fulfilled. We see Hannah praying for a son, and God granted her request.

5.      **Family influencer** – God gave women an extraordinary gift of influence. They act as a link between children and fathers and balance everyone. When Fathers become tough, they ensure that they convince the children that daddy doesn't hate them, but maybe it's due to their wrongs. This balances love, emotions, and discipline in the children.

On the contrary, we have encountered cases where foolish women turn children against their fathers, planting a seed of hatred in them. This is calling a direct curse on your children. No matter how wicked their father is, teach them to respect and love him. - *Proverbs 17:1*

6.      **Maintains a friendly home atmosphere** – The woman determines the atmosphere, the mood, and how things will run at home. If she nags or quarrels, the home becomes a little hell. They maintain joy, happiness, order, and peace.  They make a home an inhabitable place to dwell.

*Psalms 128:3 Your wife shall be like a fruitful vine in the very heart of your house, your children will be like olive plants round about your table.*

The right atmosphere will usher God's presence into your home, while the wrong atmosphere attracts the devil and his activities, which will bring torment.

**Word of advice:** Apply the same systems of teaching and instructions to avoid conflicts, comparison, gaps, and confusion in children.

**Word of advice:** Apply the same systems of teaching and instructions to avoid conflicts, comparison, gaps, and confusion in children.

> *Apply the same systems of teaching and instructions to avoid conflicts, comparison, gaps and confusion in children.*

# Chapter 6

## The Untold Truth of Children Raised in Family Crisis

The family structure has recently changed, and children are raised in different family setups. This includes single parenthood (single father and mother) mainly due to divorce or cohabitation; blended families where parents come with children from previous relationships and form a family unit; others are raised by their grandmothers in the village while their mother is in town.

Statistics show that nearly 45% of children are not living with their biological parents, which is a threat to our children, traditional values, and Godly families. The mindset of what constitutes a nuclear family is dying off; especially among women who are now more educated and have money and careers. We have met several women with 3 to 4 children from different fathers, and each father takes care of their child. One said it's a modern way of doing things and getting money, especially when all their fathers support them. However, problems arise when one father refuses to take responsibility, which confuses that child while the other kids receive gifts and support from their father.

Therefore, this has changed the face of parenting and contributed to both crisis and success in children, which we have experienced firsthand creating gaps and confusion in children. God intends for us to raise children in a nuclear family of father and mother to instill Godly family values in them, which have changed today. This has created a rise in single parenthood, where over 65% of children are being raised by their mother and 4% by their father. Consideration that, this menace is creating more harm to our children, which has been clearly shown due to the rise of teenage parenthood, come-we-stay marriages, mental health issues, drug abuse, polygamy, and divorces. The family value is declining.

Earlier on, we stated that children are fruits and rewards of marital covenant. Everyone dreams of getting married and having children in a nuclear family. However, along the way, this dream may get aborted.  At a tender age, many young people engage in sexual relationships which often results to unplanned children. The situation forces this father to abandon the child since the responsibilities are too much, and probably he is not ready to settle down.  Others are forced to get married to avoid societal shame, and after some time, they break up.  At a tender age, this girl is frustrated, broken, and left with a child to take care of with no source of income. The question is, how will this girl take care of this child soberly in this valley of confusion? Secondly, who will marry this girl with a child? And even if it happens, will this new partner give this child a decent upbringing? Consequently, do you think this runaway father will succeed after abandoning his blood? Also, what's the fate of this child?

This is where the foundations are destroyed and single motherhood and absentee fatherhood automatically sets in. After some years, this girl will get married or probably remain single, which means this child will be raised either in a broken home, in single motherhood, or by relatives, especially the grandmother, which is unfair. Therefore, this will address how crisis of families impacts children, which has become a menace in our society. This menace can be avoided through intentional parenting.

As we address this, Jane remembers being raised by her single mum, who struggled to provide for them, it was not a walk in the park; it had a myriad of challenges. Single parenthood has become embraced today and is almost an acceptable norm in our modern society.

This has seen stellar efforts towards girl child empowerment and independence amongst women, which has changed the perspective of parenting, terming single motherhood as fashionable.

Phrases like *'single by choice'* or *'what a man can do, a woman can do better'* have been adopted to strengthen this agenda. Almost every birth certificate bears the mother's name, showing absentee fatherhood.

Today, an independent woman only needs a man to give her a child. But the truth is, the devil plans to fight the agenda of a Godly family. *1 Corinthians 7:8-9, To the unmarried and the widows, I say it is good for them to remain single, as I am. But if they cannot exercise self-control, they should marry. For it is better to marry than to burn with passion".*

Paul talks of celibacy, which is singlehood by serving God, not the singleness we see today. It's no longer single by serving GOD but due to sexual sin, which is the story of many people that can be avoided. From the beginning of

*Genesis 2:18, God created everything and termed it good, only for man not to leave alone.* And that's why He created a help mate (**Genesis 2:18**).

In *Genesis 21:8-9,* We see God disregarding Ishmael, the son of Abraham, and Hagar, the mistress, and regards Isaac as the sole heir.

We tend to believe that these children are born under a spiritual fight, and that's why the majority end up struggling with curses in their lives. We don't refute single mothers raise outstanding children, but it's not easy, especially for children and also for them.

The reason behind the boy-child crisis is that boys are not raised to be real men in this generation. They copy everything they grow up seeing their mother practice, like plaiting their hair, piercing, and doing pedicures and manicures.

*Outcomes of broken families to children.*

1. These children may likely to suffer from social, emotional, and economic setbacks. Many may lack basic needs, drop out of school, lack a sense of direction, face rejection, and lack guidance and modeling. Statistically, 71% of high school dropouts in Kenya are raised in fatherless homes,

while 35% are less likely to drop out in a home with two parents.
To survive, the majority of these mothers are forced to look for men to help them pay for the expenses, which has led to these children becoming physically, emotionally, and sexually abused by these men.

2.  These children lack the bigger picture of a healthy family and marriage since they never grew up with their father and mother. A majority of them end up being divorced due to a lack of proper training on how to build a home or due to generational spirits.

3. Additionally, you deny them fatherly or motherly love, care, training, security, and identity. This is especially true in single-parenting, blended, and abandoned homes. These children are perceived as bastards and outcasts.

4. You raise half-baked men who are soft and tender and who are not taught to take responsibility as men. In marriage, they wait for their wives to bring food into the house since, all along; they grew up seeing their mother bringing food. Many copy their mother's girlish behavior, like plaiting hair, piercing ears, and other body piercings.

5. They suffer emotional emptiness and battle with feelings of abandonment and rejection. Children feel their father never wanted anything to do with them. Even if they

become raised in another family, they feel that's not their root, and many resolve to trace their roots to fill the vacuum. Many, especially boys, result to drug abuse and criminality. 85% of children in prisons come from fatherless homes.

6. They develop behavioral and emotional challenges like bitterness, aggression, and depression. No one is there to teach boys how to become responsible men with authority and good leadership to have a stable family in the future. This is the reason behind runaway fathers who have no value for children and families.

For the girls, there is no one to teach them how to become marriageable women, and despite having a promising career and money, they lack the value of a wife. These women possess an independent and defensive mentality which cripples their submissive role in marriage and ends up controlling their husbands. Many ends up divorced due to a lack of training in running a home. 71% of teenage mothers emanate from single mothers' homes.

7. When these children, especially in single-parenthood families, see you struggling to make ends meet, they feel the burden is too much for you. Sometimes, they lack basic needs like education and only wish that mum had a helper. Some children resolve to work and assist in playing their absentee father's responsibilities. A boy once confessed to

selling drugs in school to support her mother when his dad was trapped in alcoholism.

8. Many end up traumatized, primarily due to society's stigma, being shamed by other kids at school. Also, this trauma can emanate from the other siblings, especially in blended families, if this child finds out that's not their original root. We have heard rivalry, hate, and jealousy among these children, and some have even killed themselves due to mental pressure. 63% of youth suicides emanate from fatherless homes.

A very sexually active generation with loose moral values has arisen. This has led to the engagement of sexual relations at a very tender age, breeding all forms of perversion, including LGBTQ, incest, and fornication. These relationships have brought forth many children, and the cycle continues. This is a trap that the devil is using to finish the families. Therefore, we should embark on a journey to caution our children against this crisis and assist them in having happy marriage by strengthening home training. Instead, we should not sit and watch our generation go into ruins. The only genuine reason for being single should be the death of a spouse or marital abuse that has resulted in divorce.

This is the deal: despite which state you may be, either single, divorced, or remarried, remember the promises of God, that those who know the Lord can take comfort in

recognizing that they are never alone. God promises to be a father to the fatherless and a defender of widows and orphans (**Psalm 68:5**). Undertake the assignment with full Armor but prevent the same life from being replicated in your children. It's not easy.
**Solutions to this crisis.**

**1. Mend the foundation by Serving God and rooting yourself and your children in God** - this is the foundation of raising a Godly generation full of blessings. As long as they are in Christ, the benefits of redemption become their right. Today, this is the secret behind the success of many single mothers' children. If the world throws you, throw yourself to God, and you can never go wrong. Godly children will follow the systems of God; hence, God will ensure they marry right and raise Godly offspring.

**2. Show them the right path to follow.**
In cases where singlehood or divorce was caused by marital breakup or sexual sin, it is essential to address this issue with your children to admonish them not to emulate the same lifestyle.

A good majority married the wrong partners whom they never intended but were forced by circumstances, monetary gain, fame, and class.

This, therefore, necessitates a value system of a Godly marriage be inculcated in them so that there would be a desire to look forward to glorious weddings.

Our parents desired this, and by God's grace, we walked down the aisle and we are happily married. This will help them shun away from fornication, respect their bodies, and preserve themselves till marriage.

## 3. Tell your children the truth that this crisis is against God's plan.

God's plan for marriage right from creation was pure. It was meant for companionship, happiness, joy, and laughter. Therefore, any crisis is against the will of God, and hence, you should wage war against satanic forces against you.

*Isaiah 42:22-25 But this is a people robbed and spoiled; they are all of them snared in holes, and they are hid in prison houses: they are for a prey and none delivereth; for a spoil, and none saith, Restore.*

Therefore, let them know that living as a single parent or divorcee is not a lifestyle to be desired. It is riddled with all manner of ills and pains, such as loneliness, never-ending struggles, emptiness, lack of essential commodities, societal stigma, disrespect, and broken hearts.

This struggle is avoidable; hence, you should raise them to be marriageable girls and boys. Imagine if these two Godly people with the same goals marry; they will raise exceptional children full of life. Despite having success and money, many single parents are unhappy, especially in their old age.

**4. Break that cycle of singlehood, divorce, and marital conflicts within your generation together.**

This menace can be generational, and many people have traced specific patterns within their families that occur perpetually, like divorces, getting children out of wedlock, and general stagnation.  In Genesis, we trace the generation of Abraham who slept with Hagar, a servant being replicated when his grandson Jacob's wife Rachael gave him a servant, Bilhah (**Genesis 30:5**), to bear him a son when she was challenged with barrenness like Sarah.

Therefore, be cautious and break every yoke of singlehood and divorce and plant an altar of Godly marriages in the life of your children. Let the children be aware and fight battles with revelation. This is what worked for us. The moment we traced a pattern of broken homes within our families, we resolved to research what constitutes a Godly home. We waged good warfare against the hindrances prayerfully, and God blessed our reunion.

*Colossians 2:15 And having disarmed the powers and authorities, he made a public spectacle of them, triumphing over them by the cross.*

**5. Package your children with good morals and values** to respect their bodies and themselves.

*Romans 12:1 Therefore, I urge you, brothers and sisters, in view of God's mercy, to offer your bodies as a living sacrifice, holy and pleasing to God—this is your true and proper worship.*

This will help them not to waste their precious lives with meaningless relationships but rather to serve God and focus on their careers.  Let no man make them mothers before becoming wives. Let them marry Godly partners of their choice to avert all this crisis. Your children shall be preserved in Jesus' name.

**6. Set family culture, taboos, and code of conduct that governs your home.**

These are dos and don'ts that each family must have. This helps the children from taming their sexual appetites. Teach them and create a desire for them to have homes. For example, no one should ever get children out of wedlock.

In *Deuteronomy 22:22-27* according to Jewish traditions, fornication was forbidden, and once caught, it was punishable by death. We have seen families benefiting from this culture, ensuring all children are born and brought up in a complete family setup.

**7. Look for father figures to help you mentor your children.** These can be uncles, brothers-in-law, grandfathers, and pastors. These people should have godly morals that can impact life for these children. This is especially true for a boy child who is in crisis today. Let them be taught the values, traditions, and culture of being a man. Single motherhood has contributed to raising half-baked men who have no regard for family and children. Many are plaiting hair, putting up makeup, staying and being fed by women, staying at home playing video games, and waiting for women to bring food. This is a lack of proper training; that will give rise to morally upright children who will not engage in deranged behaviors and waste their precious bodies.

**8. Get married to a Godly man who will help you raise your children in a Godly manner.**

Go back to God's original design as stated in Psalms *11:3: If the foundations be destroyed, what can the righteous do?*

Marry a Christian man and raise children together, as stated in *2 Corinthians 6:14-18.* **Be *ye not unequally yoked together with unbelievers: for what fellowship hath*** *righteousness with unrighteousness? And what communion hath light with darkness?*

It is also vital to cautiously and carefully involve your children in this process. A Godly man will help instill marriage instincts in your children through perfect example.

*1 Timothy 5:14-15* gives a discrete solution to all single people. Young people are admonished to marry and get children, but if it's impossible to get married, then devote your life to Jesus and His service in the house of God. Contrary, if you have the grace to stay celibate you will find peace and satisfaction.

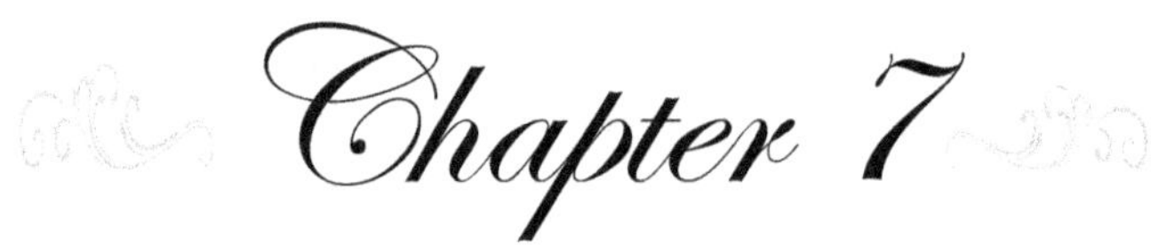

# Chapter 7

## Dragon killing the purpose and power of men

I hear a voice from afar, whispering but in deep groans, seeking for help. It's a desperate voice of a boy child. We are living in a world where the girl child is empowered economically and career-wise to a point where the world thinks that they don't need a man. Just walk into a bank or a big company, and you will realize ladies are the majority, but men are standing in the doorway as soldiers. Women also work in male-dominated jobs like construction sites, driving, quarries, engineering, and surveys.

But the big question is, what is the bigger picture behind this empowerment? Is it because men are lax, and women are forced to be empowered to cover up their responsibilities and escape from men's frustrations? Who is training the man to live with this empowered woman to perceive them as an asset, not as a threat? It's a considerable controversy. The fact is that the boy's child is in crisis.

The war against the male gender began in the bible. We see several occasions when the killing of the male gender was authorized.

*Exodus 1:22 And Pharaoh charged all his people, saying, Every son that is born ye shall cast into the river, and every daughter ye shall save alive.*

*Numbers 31:17 Now therefore kill every male among the little ones and kill every woman that hath known man by lying with.*

*Deuteronomy20:13 And when the LORD your God delivers it into your hands, you shall strike every male in it with the edge of the sword.*

*In **Mathew 2:13-18**,* Herod plotted to eliminate the messiah, the savior, the liberator. This clearly shows that the salvation of humankind could have been interfered with, but the good news is that God's plan had to be accomplished according to the prophecies. God was keen on the male child – the seed- from creation. In *Revelation 12:1-7* we see how the devil waged war against this pregnant woman (church), but God's purpose was that this male child (Jesus) would shepherd all nations.

we think that even today, the devil is very calculative and wants to finish the star, the liberator, and the head – the man. This is by attacking their voice, influence, and leadership and finally putting them to the grave. The bigger picture is to destroy the family, church, society and the entire world.

The man is the seed carrier, and if you want to finish a generation, begin from the head. The devil is determined to finish families by reorganizing the order of God, where man is the head.

*Ephesians 5:23 For the husband is the head of the wife even as Christ is the head of the church, his body, and is himself the Savior.*

Once the families are attacked, the church of Christ is affected. And he is succeeding. Just look at churches; men who are the head are very few, only to find them in bars and entertainment joints.

The foundation of manhood is not only about having money or successful careers but also the essence of being subject to the maker's authority, who will help them lead the family and the church. We see wealthy, influential, and successful men with broken families living very miserable lives and end up dying with regrets, leaving their children fighting for properties.

Today's parenting isn't the earlier one where fathers were dictators and ruthless, and children adopted. A girl resolved to run away from home due to family conflicts. In the process, she was lured by a man, and due to the desperate situation, she gave in and was defiled. After a long tussle, she came for counseling. After she narrated her story, we asked her, who wronged you? She said my father because he doesn't love me, he abuses me, and he is so harsh on me and mum too. She said she has fears once she goes to a school far away, her father will hurt her mum.

This is how fear-based parenting has been replaced with soft parenting with balanced reasoning, training, and discipline. Today, look at homes where fathers are present; they have become lions, very tough and unapproachable to their children. They only pay bills but have no connection or modeling to children. Children fear and vanish at their appearance, bringing a disconnection.

The Bible talks of restoring children to their father, which connotes a disconnection.

*Malachi 4:6 And he shall turn the heart of the fathers to the children, and the heart of the children to their fathers, lest I come and smite the earth with a curse.*

Therefore, to restore families, begin by restoring the boy child. That's why there is a parenting crisis, whereby a breed of men has emerged in the 21st century due to poor parenting.

**These are traps that the devil is using to sweep out men.**

*The Spirit of Lust.*

Sex is spiritual; sex doesn't only destroy the body, but it's a medium of transference of spirits, which destroys destinies and dreams. Women have brought down many men. This comes when the spirit of whoredoms invades their lives, diverting them from their families and serving God.

*Hosea 5:4. "Their deeds do not permit them to return to their God. A spirit of prostitution is in their heart; they do not acknowledge the LORD.*

This generation has glorified and indulged in sexual relations with same-sex relatives, rape, and animals. Some have side chicks because they have no control over their sexual urges. Out of every ten cases that we handle, five cases emanate from sexually perverted practices.

Women have destroyed kings. An example is King David, who committed adultery with Bathsheba when other men were in battle. *2 Samuel 11:1-2*. He paid a very hefty price for this iniquity since we trace his son Amnon raping Tamar, her sister (**2 Samuel 13:14**). Consequently, his son Solomon turned to idol worship influenced by strange women that he married. This is why, in **Proverbs 31:3**, Solomon warns his son against investing strength and money in women.

My spiritual mentor, Pastor Amani, says that strange women have the power to turn a powerful man into an ordinary biscuit (*Proverbs 6:26*)

Sacred sex has lost meaning. Casual sex is found everywhere, even with no struggle, putting men at risk. All you need to do is throw a few coins, and girls will come running. Once you walk in the streets, women dress seductively and naked. In beauty parlors and barber shops, these girls are parading themselves with services to entice men. And since men awaken their emotions via sense of sight, many

> *A strange woman has the power to turn a powerful man into an ordinary biscuit.*

have fallen victim proving these are end times that were prophesied.

*Isaiah4:1; and in that day seven women will take hold of one man and say, "We will eat our own food and provide our own clothes; only let us be called by your name. Take away our disgrace!"*

Standing in a bus park we saw a young man driving a Mercedes Benz. Two girls close to us whispered, "See that ride, and she shouted to him, hi! Nice car." Immediately, the guy stopped and picked up the girls. We asked ourselves, are they not strangers? Does anyone have an idea whether the other one can harm them? We realized any man who shows signs of money, success, and direction is a target.

Sex has been commercialized. Sex is being used for ritual and witchcraft purposes. That's why we hear news of girls being killed and their body parts taken. It is an open secret that some men depend on rich women for survival. Their work is to enhance their looks and muscles in gyms and beauty parlous to entice women in exchange for money. This has swept men's strength, position, voice, glory, and wisdom.  Real men of courage and character are fading off gradually, and drastic measures should be taken right from the family level.

Look at Samson; he revealed the secret of his strength to Delilah, who destroyed him, *Judges 16:17-19*. A generation of 'Delilah 'like women have risen who have no regard for family and are only interested in money gains. They don't care whether you are married; they will lure you to their chamber and trap you in an evil relationship.

In contrast, we see men like Joseph in *Genesis 39:9, 21* who refused to yield to the demands of his master's wife. God used him to preserve Israel.

*1 Corinthians 6:9, or do you not know that wrongdoers will not inherit the kingdom of God? Do not be deceived: Neither the sexually immoral nor idolaters nor adulterers nor men who have sex with men.*

Every man who escaped this vicious trap became a generational changer. We declare that your boys will not be trapped in this menace in Jesus' name.

## Abandoning Family and Children

This is a breed of men who sired children before or in marriage and abandoned their fatherhood responsibilities having no regard or value for the family and leaving all responsibilities to the women.

This commonly happens when frustrations and disagreements set in; they resolve to cowardly run away to avoid facing their misdeeds or disappointments, leaving their wife and children behind. Consequently, this leads to more frustration.

How many men have been trapped and found themselves with two or more wives simply because they disagreed with the first wife? When responsibilities and demands increase, these men run to an unknown island to escape pressure. Their children are somewhere crying and struggling out of abandonment, battling with life alone with no pillar to hold on or model to pattern after.

The scripture cannot be broken; what a man sows is what he reaps. These men plant wrong seeds and receive due punishment from the righteous judge of all, the Lord God. Mostly, nothing they endeavor to do bring forth fruits; they put in sweat and blood with no tangible results.

*Proverbs 11:29He that troubles his own house shall inherit the wind: and the fool shall be a servant to the wise of heart.*

In the Jewish tradition, any man caught having sexual intercourse with a virgin was forced to pay the bride price *Exodus 22:16*. Every action is a seed, and the harvest shall surely mature. The evil you plant will come back a hundredfold.

> *He that troubles his own house shall inherit the wind.*

*Luke 6:38 Give, and it will be given to you: good measure, pressed down, shaken together, and running over will be put into your bosom. For with the same measure that you use, it will be measured back to you."*

In the end, these men die a very miserable life out of frustration, especially in old age, for disregarding the commands of God on parenting.

## The Addict.

This is a cluster of men who, as a result of reckless living and pursuit of fantasy, have surrounded their lives with the drunkenness of alcohol and hard drugs as an escape route to the realities of life.

It probably began as fun with friends as a result of peer or parental influence, and addiction creped in slowly. They are the party bad boys 'who take life as fanfare and are never serious. They move from one place to another, clubbing and holding parties at the expense of their lives. This has taken away their dreams, destinies, purpose, visions, homes, voices, and influence, and poverty crisp in like an armed robber.

*Proverbs 23:21 For the drunkard and the glutton will come to poverty, and drowsiness will clothe a man with rags.*

They have abandoned their family responsibilities since they are unproductive.

*Proverbs 20:1 Wine is a mocker; strong drink is raging: whosoever is deceived is not wise.*

When children are left under the care of their mothers to train and model without a father's input, they often resent the father figure. Therefore, men who practice these uncouth tendencies only reap disrespect and frustration from their children.

Noah, in **Genesis9:21-24,** disgraced himself in front of his sons. The contrast in **Genesis 19:30-38**isan account of how the daughters of Lot intoxicated him with wine with the intent to have sexual intercourse with him one at a time and ended up siring the Moabite tribe. *Luke 21:34*says that drunkenness is a trap and a destroyer.

Walk along the streets, especially behind uncompleted buildings; men sit chewing khat and bhang while women are in their businesses making money. What about rehabilitation centers? Men are the majority.

What pains me most is how the devil has blinded these men to the point of defending their indulgence in wine and illicit addictions, that wine is good for the stomach.

The big question that should be on everyone's mind is: what sort of joy can be derived from imbibing such things that cause paralysis both in the body and mind to the point of total dysfunctionality? It should be known by now that reaching this level is no longer fun. It is a menace.

We have seen men selling properties at a throwaway price only to drink all the money to the detriment of their families.

One girl came crying since she passed her exams so well, but her father couldn't afford her school fees. Why? He had sold all his inherited land and finished the money in drinking dens. This girl was so bitter and wounded, and she can't be blamed; everybody would be, too. Do you think if this girl, by God's grace, goes to the university, gets a good job, and becomes successful, she will come and appreciate her father? It's impossible. She will give him coins and lavish thousands of goodies to the mother who took care of her. This is not the devil; it's the fruits of what you planted. Fathers, let's be wise.

## Spirit of Heaviness.

In our times, men need to be psychologically strong enough to handle pressure. The male gender is endangered from all corners. The man is at the center of the family, work, community, money, career, responsibilities, wife, children, in-laws, and the whole clan.  Balancing all this angers them, especially if they lack support.

The spirit of heaviness is behind this turmoil after stealing men's joy, hope, and faith. It covers them with a cloud of confusion, agitation, and mental turmoil. And many find it difficult to confide and share their struggles. Sin is also a contributing factor, and that's why they attract affliction since they lost their identity in God.

**Zephaniah** *1:17I will bring such distress on all people that they will grope about like those who are blind because they have sinned against the* LORD. *Their blood will be poured out like dust and their entrails like dung.*

When a man is distressed, they exhibit animosity by fighting or running away, which shows an inability to handle frustrations healthily. News of men committing suicide and murder are always on top of almost every broadcast. Behind the killings lies a frustrated man.  A case we dealt with of a man in distress who was on the verge of killing his ex-wife. He married her when she already had two children, and after raising them on his own, she eloped with another man. All his life resources and efforts were wasted, and he felt used. Sadly later, he committed suicide due to frustration.

God desires to restore every broken spirit and anoint men with the oil of gladness.

*Isaiah 61:3 to appoint unto them that mourn in Zion, to give unto them beauty for ashes, the oil of joy for mourning, the garment of praise for the spirit of heaviness; that they might be called trees of righteousness, the planting of the LORD, that he might be glorified.*

## Pride.

Pride is having a sense of self-importance, a superior mindset, and a negative ego. Pride is the biggest destroyer.

Society regards manhood as being self-reliant prowess in their minds and actions, which keeps them from asking for help when, in fact, they desperately need it. The ego in men has yet to accept that they are lagging, and a lot of efforts required empowering themselves. Look at many institutions; men are the bosses and CEOs, but all other employees are women. Many men possess pride, arrogance, and wrong attitude, which is a cancer to destiny. It's difficult for a man to accept help from another man. - *Proverbs 27:17*

Previously, we heard one family member confronting his well-up brother, who supported him in setting up a business simply because he corrected him. Currently the man closed the business thinking that his brother hates him and as we write this book, the 45-year-old man is in the village being fed by his mother and unable to educate his children. Untamed ego is dangerous which is the reason behind the frustration of many men.

Most egoistic men will never accept defeat, even when it is obvious to everyone else. It's difficult for some men to admit that they are down and struggling, which has made them fall behind, especially in this era where women are dominating. They are over confident in their abilities and potential.  This breeds pride, a superior mindset, and arrogance, which creates havoc on their relationships, personal development, and connections. A negative ego has destroyed families and brought about dictatorship, abuse, and toxic masculinity. Being the family leader and provider gives these men the audacity to do what they want.

Allowing pride to thrive and grow makes them arrogant, narrow-minded, and stubborn. All of this limits their potential. It's common to see a young, broke man disrespecting his boss and walking out of employment simply because they have been corrected. That's why many men lack favor, and poverty is eating them up.

In **1 Peter 5:5**God calls us to humility and will lift us; men are called to gentleness, patience, and self–control by exhibiting biblical masculinity (rooted in Christ). Jesus is a perfect example of a person who was resilient in pursuing

God, gentle in spirit, and humble in serving others. - **Galatians 5:22-23**

We have encountered humble men enjoying favor and job opportunities from other men by humility and honoring them. I declare that a negative ego will not hinder the progress of your boys in Jesus 'name.

*James 4:6-7 But he gives us more grace. That is why Scripture says: "God opposes the proud but shows favor to the humble.*

**The spirit of mammon.**

The society perceives a real man as the one endowed with money. Any man with money earns power, voice, respect, and influence. The Bible alludes in *Ecclesiastes7:12That wisdom is a defense, and money is a defense.*

The bible does not discourage being wealthy, it gives us wisdom on prioritizing God at the expense of money **Mathew 6: 33**. Everyman focus should be placing God at the center of his pursuit and money is an addition. The love of money is idolatry which offends God.

A man with true Godly character, wise but without money, gets ridiculed and disregarded and perceived not to be a real man, and his qualities are never regarded as in the case of one wise man in:-

*Ecclesiastes 9:15-16 Now there was found in it a poor wise man, and he by his wisdom delivered the city; yet no man remembered that same poor man. Then said I, Wisdom is better than strength: nevertheless, the poor man's wisdom is despised, and his words are not heard.*

To suit these expectations and the responsibilities bestowed upon men, the Love for money and the demands have pushed men to a very tight corner that they are determined to get it at any cost. This has led them to engage in criminal activities like corruption, drug trafficking, unclean business deals, witchcraft, and cultism resulting to frustrations and imprisonment.

*1 Timothy 6:10 For the love of money is the root of all evil: which while some coveted after, they have erred from the faith, and pierced themselves through with many sorrows.*

Money has given men a ticket to engage in evil activities to the point of abandoning one's faith and family. Look at the recent killings of girls since body organ trafficking has emerged. One serial killer confessed to having killed over 70 girls and sold their organs for sh.600,000. Look at deception and craftiness in some cultic churches due to riches and power. This love for money has led men to problems, including curses to their generations.

They trust in their wealth and boost in their great riches yet they cannot redeem themselves from death by paying a ransom to God. Their redemption is not rooted in money. Many have died miserably with strange diseases, curses, and punishment from God, leaving their properties benefitting other people. This spirit will not finish our men in Jesus' name.

**Lost Vision and Purpose.**

These men lack direction, vision, and purpose in life. They live and exist without anything to live for or achieve no God, conviction, or nothing. **Joel 2:28b** prophesies that when the spirit of God will be poured, older men shall dream, and young men shall see visions.

> *Habakkuk 2:2-3 And the LORD answered me, and said, Write the vision, and make it plain upon tables, that he may run that readeth it. For the vision is yet for an appointed time, but at the end, it shall speak, and not lie: though it tarry, wait for it; because it will surely come, it will not tarry.*

They work but have nothing to show for it; there are no savings or development. These men may have all the educational qualifications but lacks a sense of creativity and strength. Once they don't get a job or are laid off, they sit in the house with a remote for years, waiting for the wife to bring food. From creation, women were created to be helpers, and if they encounter a man with no vision, they tend to overtake and run all home affairs. In the process, women dominate, and these men lose their voice and influence.

Once you see a family lagging behind regarding development, Look at the man's leadership. Many are still renting houses at the age of 70years, and they are at the point where children have to buy land and build for them in future. The enemy does not fight success but kills the potential, bringing many men down.

Dreams are just dreams if they are not worked upon. Discipline, consistency, and hard work are required to achieve them. That's why many families are in financial crisis.

> **Dreams are just dreams if they are not worked upon.**

# Chapter 8

## How To Raise Boys to Be Real Men.

Raising boys to become men should start from an understanding that the devil has succeeded and is still very determined to diminish the vitality and potential of men to affect the family, church, and nation at large. This will equip parents to be intentional and open to teach their sons to overcome all these devil traps.

**Ezra 8:21** we see Ezra praying for the protection of his children because if this hedge of protection is broken, Satan will bite them.

*Ecclesiastes 10:8 b .......and whoso breaketh an hedge, a serpent shall bite him."*

There are ways in which this assignment can be done to produce outstanding results: -

## 1. Restore their lost identity.

Identity biblically refers to the truth of whom or what a person is. In **Genesis 1:27,** God created man in His own image (having God's capacity) and likeness (**spiritual connection**) to dominate his creation. The man was with God, and when he sinned, he was thrown out of the presence of God, losing his place. **Ecclesiastes *12:13 states that man must fear God and keep* his commands.** Today, many men have lost their place in God, like Adam in the Garden of Eden.

*Genesis. 3:17 And unto Adam he said, because thou hast hearkened unto the voice of thy wife, and hast eaten of the tree, of which I commanded thee, saying, Thou shalt not eat of it: cursed is the ground for thy sake; in sorrow shalt thou eat of it all the days of thy life.*

Therefore, God cursed the ground when man sinned, and he said that sorrow would accompany his bread. Thus, in his sinful nature, this man is a candidate for sorrow. This explains why many men have nothing to show in their sinful toil all day and night. They are still under this curse. **1 Kings11:1-25** narrates how King Solomon, who was the wisest of all, was turned to idol worship by strange women.

Therefore, every liberated man who has subjected himself to God becomes exempted from this curse. By salvation, every curse was lifted by Jesus. Teach your boys that only God can restore their lost position by seeking him and subjecting themselves to help from God, their father. Raising them with this understanding will form a base of their salvation, and they will be safe since the foundation of God is sure having the seal, the lord knoweth them who are his. (**2 timothy 2:19**)

### 2. Create a road map of mentorship.
Mentorship means discipleship. It's a process of guiding and helping another person to support their personal development. It simply means training. Fathers, your presence is the best book for your boys to read at home. Actions speak louder.

*Titus2:7 and you yourself must be an example to them by doing good works of every kind. Let everything you do reflect the integrity and seriousness of your teaching.*

This entails treating your wife with respect and honor and supporting her to achieve her dream together as a family, and this will impact the same values in your boy. Mothers help your husband's model the behavior they desire in their sons, such as respect, love, kindness, and care.

This is the main problem that has contributed to the boy-child crisis. Boys have become unruly due to a lack of mentorship from fathers at home and in society. Fathers are either absent, drunkards, violent, bitter, and irresponsible, which passively inspires the same behavioral patterns in their sons. A child is a mirror; they fashion depending on what you have trained them. And the truth is if you discover you have a breadcrumb on your lip, you don't wipe the mirror but yourself.

That is the starting point. Create avenues of mentorship by watching programs together, training them on work, attending seminars on various issues affecting them, or letting a spiritual authority speak over their life and walk the journey together with them. This will eliminate 70% of deviant behaviors in boys, like drug abuse, fornication, crime, aggression, anger, and bitterness.

### 3. Change of mindset.
Mindset is the engine and control valve of everything in life. This journey should begin by separating the truth from

fiction. It's a process of renewing and repositioning to possess.

The renewal of our minds allows us to set our thoughts and affections right and correct every misconception about life.

*Romans 12:2 And be not conformed to this world: but be ye transformed by the renewing of your mind, that ye may prove what is that good, and acceptable, and perfect, will of God.*

This involves accepting the reality that the world has changed and men are disadvantaged over women. And the bitter truth is that women are using men to empower themselves. In many companies, many men are the bosses, but 80% of employees are women. In relationships, men are the financers who change the standards of women.

In his book 'Mental Shift,' Rev. Peter Jacks puts it this way;" At the core of every great achievement lies a pivotal transformation—a profound shift in perspective, mindset, and perception. A change of perspective unlocks the latent potential within you to transcend limitations and harness your mind's transformative power".

The need for mental fortitude and resilience has never been more pronounced in a world teeming with distractions, self-doubt, and external pressures. Yet, amidst the chaos lies a reservoir of untapped potential waiting to be unleashed.

That's why many are into debt simply because they want to yield to the demands of their wives or family members. They take a loan knowing that it will be difficult for them to pay. Often you can see students working hard to pay school fees or pocket money for their girlfriends, which they cannot keep. This means their minds are set on pleasing women and society to prove they are real men. And their mind needs to be sober and smart. Teach your sons to become smart mentally to avoid being taken advantage of.

Secondly, many men possess the wrong mindset about themselves. Men care for everyone, and they forget themselves or become the last priority. They should also be aware that they are human beings who deserve care.

A while back, we visited a particular city looking for a men's collection shop since we needed stuff for my husband. We visited over 15 shops, but to my surprise, men's stuff was very scarce to the point we didn't find anything suitable. We discussed that men buy clothes and other things for the family but forget themselves. It is high time we teach our boys that self-love is not an option but essential for them. They give so much, expecting much, too, and if that doesn't work out, many end up depressed. That's why you see men killing women aimlessly due to frustrations.

My husband often say it is not simple to be a man because

> *It's not simple to be a man because everything about men is exaggerated.*

everything about men is exaggerated, including their costly clothing, work, and responsibilities. Therefore, they must fight through life situations to achieve by thinking outside the box and doing extraordinary work. The reality is that men need rescue, but if we begin training them from home, we shall raise boys who have a future of becoming mature men who will stand up for God and their families. Who will live in reality and not fake life to fit society's standards? Men who will love themselves first pursue their God-given purpose for themselves and their families. Also, men who will not be consumed with worry, anxiety, and stress about earthly things but set their minds above

*Colossians 3:2. Set your affection on things above, not on things on the earth."*

## 4. Empower their authority

Authority is the power to influence and command. The president of a nation has authority over the affairs of the country, guided by the rule of law. Therefore, man was given authority to dominate over God's creation in **Genesis** *1:28.* This authority is superior. It shows how God was so mindful of man to grant him such power to the point David in

***Psalms 8: 4-9*** was surprised to the point of questioning God. Therefore, authority is vital in God's eyes. Despite a change in modern civilization, God never changes. His word is settled forever.

*Isaiah 40:8 the grass withered, the flower fadeth: but the word of our God shall stand forever."*

The moment you change the order of God, it breeds crisis. The strength of a man does not lie in his deep voice and broad chest but in the accomplishment of the purpose God gave them (dominion). It is in the ability to submit to the authority and do the will of his God. This authority was taken by sin, but Jesus restored it.

*John 10:10he thief cometh not, but for to steal, and to kill, and to destroy: I am come that they might have life and that they might have it more abundantly."*

Sin sinks authority and power in men, which is seen in failed families, churches, and institutions. Man requires restoration of authority to rule over his domain, build his home, labor for his needs, and overcome forces against his excellent living. When a man has authority in God, every other living thing submits willingly.

> *Sin sinks authority and power in men.*

A generation of weak men has emerged, including young people who are fainting and growing weary, as prophesied in the bible. However, the solution remains on God's side since he is the giver and sustainer of strength and power to work.

*Isaiah 40:29-31He giveth power to the faint; and to them that have no might he increaseth strength." Even the youths shall faint and be weary, and the young men shall utterly fall:" But they that wait upon the LORD shall renew their strength; they shall mount up with wings as eagles; they shall run, and not be weary; and they shall walk, and not faint*

Therefore, teach your boys this concept. Then, proceed to train them to be hard, strong physically, emotionally, spiritually, and psychologically to fulfill their assignment and remain in control. In this generation, you can't afford to raise weak men. This involves subjecting themselves to God to preserve their authority. *Philippians 4:13*This will ensure they achieve everything through Christ, who gives them strength.

### 5.	Teach them their Responsibilities.  (numbering)

Responsibility is having an obligation, control, or care over something or someone as part of his role. Any education minister in a country handles issues concerning children's education in school as expected by the president. From creation, man was given the responsibility as steward of God's creation and care, and protection to his household, and whoever goes against this is termed an infidel *1 Timothy 5:8*.

This concept has been misinterpreted since this does not mean that man was given the responsibility over the extended family, the clan, and the community. Therefore, this responsibility should be defined and constrained to the immediate family. Men have become like donkeys carrying burdens to the point of being worn out. This burden should be offloaded off men's shoulders. Many men don't run away from their responsibility because they want to but because they are overburdened.

That's the bigger picture; hence, they should be packaged to undertake these roles with faithfulness. The bottom line is that boys should be taught to be responsible for their God, lives, family, and community.  Being responsible gives, you favor, blessings, and a good name in the community. Real men take up responsibilities without avoiding or delegating.

## 6. Train on Leadership traits.
Myles Monroe said that genuine leadership is one literal disposition related to one sense of purpose, self-worth, and self-concept. Leadership is not opportunistic or by chance

but a spirit in a man from God that brings understanding and inspiration.

*Job 32:8But there is **a spirit in man: and the inspiration of the Almighty giveth them understanding."***

Authentic leadership is a product of inspiration, not manipulation. It's cultivated and trained.

God bestows man as the leader of the family unit, which means that preparation for this role should be taken with the utmost seriousness. Every true leader is a product of training. *Genesis 2:11-22.* If you trace the journey of Moses, he killed an Egyptian and run into hiding in a foreign land. After decades in the desert, God had matured him and enabled him to lead his people out of slavery.

> *Leadership Is not Opportunistic.*

*Numbers 27:18* God mandated Moses to make Joshua a leader (a man with God's spirit). This spirit of leadership made him lead people to the Promised Land.

A leader gives direction, vision, and a route to follow, which we see in Moses. This entails training them to make decisions for themselves independently without being influenced or swayed away. In marriages, we spot men who are indecisive in making decisions; they must consult their mothers on every issue. Some lack any opinion, forcing the wife to make decisions in the house. This has brought chaos to many homes.

Train them to always be on the steering wheel if they want to remain in control. Lead in decisions, savings, family culture, dreams, and bringing up children in consultation with the wife's help. A certain woman has a very nice, born-again, respectful, and lovely husband. Their only problem is the need for more leadership in this man. A point came, and the woman had to take up the mantle. By now, the wife has bought family land, pays school fees for the children, and is progressing to saving to build a house. But the only problem is that the man feels threatened, which is bringing chaos. The woman felt this man would make them suffer due to a lack of leadership skills. Therefore, if boys cultivate this spirit, they can take up all mantles faithfully in all spheres of life, including politics, business, homes, and church.

## 7.    Train on the value of work.

In Genesis, we see God working by creating the universe within seven days; man was placed in the Garden of Eden to work and keep it. This means God is a worker and expects us to work. Today, a sluggard microwave generation wants to live without work. We engage with married men whose parents are paying house rent and school fees for their children, and they are not crippled. In creation, God gave man work before a wife, but due to sin, he cursed the ground and said that man would toil for his daily bread. But through redemption, Jesus lifted every curse. Therefore, any sinful man is a candidate for toil, which makes them weary or tired because of a lack of produce.

**Ecclesiastes** *10:15 the labor of the foolish wearieth every one of them, because he knoweth not how to go to the city."*

*Proverbs 14:1 the fool hath said there is no God in his heart. They are corrupt, they have done abominable works, none doeth good."*

**Proverbs 13:4** *The soul of the sluggard desireth, and hath nothing: but the soul of the diligent shall be made fat."*

*Proverbs 22:29 Seest thou a man diligent in his business? He shall stand before kings; he shall not stand before mean men. "***God is against slothfulness** *Proverbs 6: 10-11 Proverbs 20:13*

Encourage your sons to have big dreams and visions. God created a fully packaged man who could care for God's creation. Pursuing Vision and purpose will attract resources and bring fulfillment, joy, happiness, and energy to rise and face tomorrow.

Let them work in farms, change bulbs, slaughter chickens, and clear bushes and water pipes etc.  This will ensure their system adapts to work, not sit all day doing nothing. You can encounter a grown-up man who calls the neighbor to slaughter a chicken for his family. This speaks a lot.

We live in a money-oriented generation and everything requires money. Men say if you want to earn respect, have a lot of money and lots of money. The world will respect you. Money will give you a voice. This is a shield, and they should be trained to earn it.

Let your boy have skills in what he is passionate about, gifted, or talented in; this will give him a purpose in life. After the education, train on how to convert it to money in the marketplace. Skill and creativity attract money. Train them that If they lose their jobs, real men don't sit in the house playing video games as they wait for women to bring food. Instead, they should go out to sell eggs and groceries and do manual jobs to feed their families.

One man confessed that his family can never go hungry, instead he better go hawking to get daily bread. That is a real man.

Teach them about meaningful labor, which brings blessings and progress.

*Proverbs 13:11Wealth gotten by vanity shall be diminished. But he that gathered by labor shall increase.*

Do you know that any wealth of a sinner will be given to the righteous? *Proverbs 13:22b.*

Let their labor be after edifying the body of Christ, serving humanity not just heaping for their personal consumption.

*Proverbs 11:4 Wealth is worthless in the day of wrath, but righteousness delivers from death.*

Our primary concern should be righteousness because, after everything, only your soul will save you from eternal death.

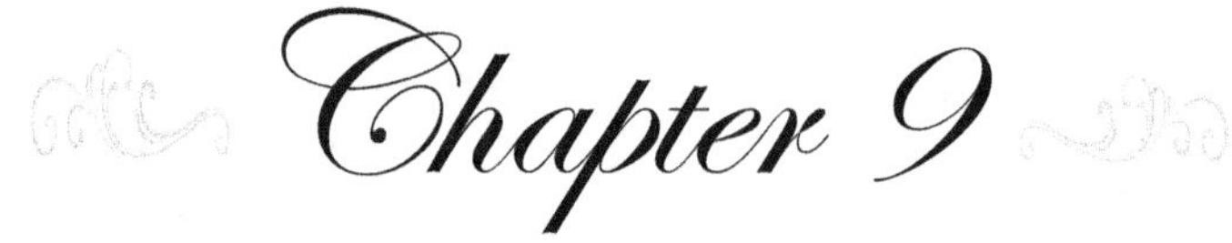

# Chapter 9

## How Negative Parenting Influences Children's Behavior.

The truth is fruits don't fall too far away from the tree. Psychologist's research show that 80% of traits children possess emanate from parental modeling.  As they grow, they pick both negative and positive behaviors. Later, as their brain develops, they process their thoughts to drop negative behaviors and learn others.

If you keenly interrogate yourself, you could identify some behaviors that you directly possessed from your parents, and over time, you have consciously passed them onto your children, too. Are you a clean freak? Are you fond of shouting at your children? Do you find yourself forcing your children to eat certain foods they don't love, especially greens, simply because you now understand their value? What about possessing some tools in the house that you probably don't use, just like your dad? The truth is all these traits were passed on from our parents.

This chapter will categorically guide you on how parenting style and skills affect the characters and traits in children.

Once again, in reference to janes case, she grew up in her grandmother's homestead with nine aunties. This meant she needed to fight for love, attention, approval, space, and survival. It was challenging to get the real culprit when anything went wrong, and sometimes everybody would point fingers at them together with her younger brother. Many times, they were innocent.

Proving a point was so difficult since nobody would listen to them. She felt harassed and angry, and defending herself was difficult.

She developed a very defensive nature; it was hard to accept simple mistakes as her responsibility, even when caught red-handed. She later realized that defensiveness is a mechanism she developed to shield herself from any pain that the effect of any accusations could cause.

She realized it was a problem when it began to cause struggles in her marriage because she defended everything, including mistakes and sound advice, to the point of not apologizing. But by the grace of God, she overcame.

Can you identify some negative behaviors you didn't love in your upbringing? That beating you received because of other people's mistake?  Being compared and expected to do like others?

The question is, how does negative parenting impact children's traits and behaviors?

**Types of bad parenting strategies.**

1. **Parents who are over-controlling.**
Just as it sounds, it refers to parents who demand blind obedience from their children without being questioned. For them, it's a do as I say affair.  They typically have stringent rules that are sometimes unreasonable and must be followed. They offer meager support but demand a high level of results in terms of behavior and performance, especially in school. They dictate every decision for their children, from the dress code, foods to eat, where to go, and

who to associate with, which robs the children's ability to think and be themselves.

When children deviate, they are given harsh punishment to control and toughen them. As a result, children grow to be unhappy, less independent, have low self-esteem, and have poor social competence. Have you ever met over-controlling people in companies, marriages, social gatherings, and churches?  These character manifestations are mainly pointers to the kind of upbringing they endured and the type of parenting they had.

A biblical example can be found in the story of King Saul in **1Samuel 20:30**. He was an angry and very threatening parent. He even hurled his spear at Jonathan, his son, to kill him. He also planned to kill David, which led to losing respect from his son.

This kind of parenting results in anti-social behavior, which happens when a person does not consider how their actions might affect others. This will eventually result when a child experiences harsher punishment and less parental warmth.

They tend to be aggressive and lack empathy, which connotes trauma. These children never experience safety and an excellent nurturing environment; hence, they use anti-social behaviors like lying, hitting, stealing, and manipulation as a defense mechanism to deal with terror and fighting. In addition, since they lack affectionate attachment to their parents, they devote themselves to provoking or frustrating the parents at every opportunity.

In adulthood, these people are aggressive towards people; they are liars and dishonest; they violate rules and are likely to be jailed; they are abusive in marriage/relationships and can abuse children, too. They mostly emit negative energy effortlessly and face a lot of rejection from society. They resolve to drug abuse and develop mental health issues like depression and anxiety. On the other hand, the opposite is true for social behaviors, which develop when a child is brought up in a warm and supportive environment.

## 2.     Parents who are lenient and over-indulgent.

This describes parents who allow their children to do whatever they wish. These parents are very loving and impose little or no rules or guidance on their children's behavior. To avoid conflict, they resolve to bribe or give privileges to them. Children make their own decisions, and parents pose more as friends to their children than authority figures. These children grow to think highly of themselves; they tend to be proud and arrogant to people and authority. They struggle to maintain relationships since they can indulge with anyone they want.

As a result, these children grow with no self-discipline; they are unruly and aggressive, especially in school, due to a lack of parental boundaries. They are poor decision makers due to lack of set guidelines, which will improve their problem-solving skills. They display low achievements in many areas since parents have little expectations for them. They live without anything to strive for.

They are the common womanizers and manipulators we spot in our society. They are unable to take responsibility for their lives and tend to turn to drug addictions due to frustrations.

We sometimes watched a billionaire empire go down the drain because of his children. This man had worked so hard to acquire many businesses, companies, assets, and millions in the accounts of his four children and their mother. After his death, the children often forcefully demanded money from their mother to go to waste. The mother was assertive and determined to protect the family property; for this reason, they saw her as a block. Therefore, they conspired and killed their mother so that they could have complete control of the inherited wealth.

Years passed, and they sold all their assets and businesses to finance their lavish lifestyle through drugs and parties.
At the time we are writing this book, two are dead; one is mentally unstable, and the other one is in jail, serving life imprisonment. This underscores a problem with improper parenting since these children were not trained to be responsible enough to carry on the legacy.

The Bible highlights the story of Eli, the priest in **1 Samuel 2:12 – 36,** who failed to order his children after it was reported to him the evil they were committing against God and the temple. His failure led to the suffering of the Israelites in **1samuel 4:10-**22 where God sent the Philistines to defeat the Israelites, and over 3000 soldiers died, including his sons. The Ark of the Covenant was also captured, which led to his death when news was brought to him.

**3. Parents who are not involved, neglectful, or absent from their children's affairs.**

Being absent takes on different dimensions; it can be emotional, physical, or geographical. This may refer to parents who don't live with their children due to work demands, divorces and conflicts. Also refers to children under the care of relatives and caregivers, abandoned children, and parents who have anti-social problems like drug addicts, mentally or physically sick, and are unable to take care of their children. These parents fail or may not provide for their children's basic needs. Children here lack emotional attachment to their parents.

Parents, in this instance, provide little or no guidance. Hence, children need help to get their way through life. These children mature very first because they resume the duties of their parents at a young age. Have you encountered a family where an underage child cooks, cleans, and cares for their siblings to the point of dropping out of school? These children tend to be unhappy, emotionally detached, have low self-esteem, and have mental health issues. Have you ever spotted a person who is always over-serious (no non-sense people as society calls them), they don't see anything funny and pleasing in life? Probably, they underwent such parenting.

A friend confessed that he never loved his father simply because he refused to take him to high school. He was forced to do manual jobs to the point of selling bhang to get school fees. After high school, by God's grace, he got a scholarship to college and later a good job. Even now, he struggles to relate with his father since he feels he has the capability but neglects his responsibilities towards him.

This implies that as a child, all his physical, emotional, love, and security needs were never met, and hence had an inner conflict.

For example, in **1 Kings 1:5- 6,** King David was a military and uninvolved man.  He failed to discipline his son Adonijah and Absalom for killing his brother Amnon who raped Tamar.

**2 Samuel 14:28,** he refused to resolve issues with Absalom after he returned to Jerusalem.

This kind of parenting results in poor resilience and low self-esteem in children who, consequently, possess a low sense of their worth and value, lacking confidence in their abilities and opinions. In adulthood, these people might become people pleasers to gain approval and, more often, are abused and taken advantage of differently.

A lady confessed to having faced a lot of punishments in childhood and was never given a chance to explain herself; she was literally abused, called names, and sexually abused by a cousin at the age of 9 years. This, as you would imagine, changed her self-perception. She has struggled to accept herself and believe in her abilities since no one was there to listen to her and appreciate her. Right now, she has three kids from 3 different relationships at 26 years old, divorced and emotionally broken. The first relationship ended as a result of infidelity, the second one left her with huge loans and debt-ridden that the spouse had borrowed in her name, and the 3rd one was very toxic and abusive; her well-being and peace was+ never considered.

After a self-worth test was carried out, she realized the guys were not the problem; herself-worth created a lot of insecurities and jealousy in her to the point she fought with her husband's colleague in front of a client in a hotel who had gone for a business deal. She never wanted anyone near her husband. She was possessive and wanted him all for herself. Also, accepting love and intimacy was a problem since she felt detached from her partner. These behaviors choked the husband to extramarital affairs, which finally led to their separation.

Often, she finds herself giving out all her salary to friends and relatives to please them. Saying no is a problem.  This tells you that parenting messed with her self-worth, and the sad part is that she finds herself being abusive to her children due to anger. This is the deal; this lady needs to go through a journey of self-acceptance to raise children with high self-worth.

In conclusion, if your child is exhibiting negative behavior, it's a sign that they haven't developed the skills to manage their emotions and has an underlying communication difficulty. These behaviors include lying, bullying, being ungrateful, disrespectful, disobedient, laziness, using foul language, greed, aggression, stealing, and refusal to go to school. Resolve to practice intentional parenting by journaling the negative behaviors and working them out. Begin by observing what you do, how you communicate, and the body language, words, and actions you exhibit to your children.

# *Chapter 10*

## Strategies for Influential and Effective Parenting

It's the joy of any parent to raise happy, disciplined, resilient, focused, and independent children. Many children are raised with little or no guidance and grow without knowing who they are and what they aspire to achieve.

Imagine a situation whereby parents identify children's potential, passion, and talents at a young age and channel their support towards that area. The results will be evident. Today, young, educated youths are idle, doing nothing simply because they lack innovative and creative skills.

Additionally, most are in the job market simply because of money, not because they enjoy what they do. What about the emotionally crippled, bitter, and mentally challenged children? This may point to misdeeds or mishaps during upbringing. These strategies will assist you in raising a happy generation mentally, spiritually, physically, socially, and emotionally.

For example, our six-year-old daughter is talented in singing, and now she has a music teacher. By ten years, she says she will be a star. we have seen this goal push her to practice more, watch kids singing in auditions and talent shows, and sing in Sunday school. Do you relate this to your upbringing? Everybody wanted to become a teacher or an accountant simply because we never knew our goals and aspirations.

Let us discuss some of the best strategies that can assist you in raising a fulfilled generation with biblical examples; you can apply the strategy co-currently or pick whatever suits your situation. But the truth is they will add value to your children's behavior.

**Spiritual strategies**

## 1.    THE WORD.

The word of God is the master key to life; it can open or lock any destiny. Everything that demands effective parenting is obtainable in the word. The word is where it all begins; it's the foundation of our knowledge and packaged in the bible, which we believe, is the safest guide to our children's destiny.

*John 1:1-3 in the beginning was the Word, and the Word was with God, and the Word was God. The same was in the beginning with God. All things were made by him, and without him was not anything made that was made*

*Colossians 1:16 For in him all things were created: things in heaven and on earth, visible and invisible, whether thrones or powers or rulers or authorities; all things have been created through him and for him.*

The word is the seed of God, which should be planted in the hearts of our children Luke *8:11-18,* which, when cultivated, can help our children bear Godly fruits. It conditions the heart to love God, and just as a seed has to remain in the ground over time to germinate, the word of God has to abide in their heart. Jesus said, **John15:7** *ye abide in me, and my words abide in you, ye shall ask what ye will, and it shall be done unto you.*

This will help them to walk in Godliness and overcome the evil patterns of this world.

According to the scriptures, all God is all His Word is. Anything that cannot stop God can't stop His Word from having its way.

**The Word creates solutions**. - During the first appearance of the Word in the creation story, it created a solution to a battered world. **Genesis 1:1-3 (See also Hebrews 1:3). In the beginning, God created the Heaven and the earth. And the earth was without form and void, and darkness was upon the face of the deep. And the Spirit of God moved upon the face of the waters. And God said, let there be light, and there was light.** Likewise, God's Word still creates solutions today. This is why when we believe in Him, His Word creates solutions for parenting by aligning them with the will of God.

We also understand that God is Spirit, and so is His Word. That means God's Spirit is domiciled in His Word. The Bible says: *God is a Spirit: and they that worship him must worship him in spirit and truth (John 4:24)*

Therefore, **the word calms the spirit of our children**. This ensures they produce and portray the fruit of the spirit in their lives, like love, joy, peace, patience, and kindness. Jesus, speaking on the potency of the Word, said:
*It is the spirit that quickeneth; the flesh profiteth nothing: the words that I speak unto you, they are spirit, and they are life (John 6:63; See also Ezekiel 2:2).*

**The word is a powerful tool of war.** The Spirit of the Lord in the Word levels every mountain of the wicked on our paths and empowers us to win the war. Therefore, when we engage the Word in the battle against our children's destiny, our triumph is guaranteed **(Zechariah 4:6-7; 2 Corinthians 2:14)**. Thus, when we say, 'It is written,' the Spirit of the Word goes forth to challenge our challengers, confront our challenges and bring us victory.

*As it is written: So, shall they fear the name of the Lord from the west, and his glory from the rising of the sun. When the enemy shall come in like a flood, the Spirit of the Lord shall lift up a standard against him (Isaiah 59:19).*

The word of God will enhance their boldness to speak against every barrier in their lives.

It is also important to note that **God's Word carries sanctifying virtues**. We understand from the scriptures that God and His Word are Holy. Thus, it cleans up and perfects the lifestyle of God's people.

The Bible says: *Wherewithal shall a young man cleanse his way? by taking heed thereto according to thy word. Thy word have I hid in mine heart, that I might not sin against thee (Psalms 119:9, 11; See also 1 Peter 1:16).*

This is why when the Word of God comes alive in us, we become naturally sanctified.

*John 17:17 Sanctify them through thy truth: thy word is truth. (It is also written: Now ye are clean through the word which I have spoken unto you (John 15:3).*

This virtue of unrighteousness has destroyed this generation; sin is a destroyer.

When God's word enters their hearts, it will make your children prosperous. Teach them day and night.

*Joshua 1:8 This book of the law shall not depart out of thy mouth; but thou shalt meditate therein day and night, that thou mayest observe to do according to all that is written therein: for then thou shalt make thy way prosperous, and then thou shalt have good success.*

Every negative behavior portrays a lack of the word of God in our children's hearts—any rudeness, envy, hate, and ungodliness. For out of the abundance of the heart, the mouth speaks. **Proverbs 4:23**

## 2.      PRAYER.

Prayer is vital to unleashing God-given destiny in our children based on his word. It involves giving thanks to God for our children and aligning their lives, destiny, behavior, health, and salvation in the altar of prayer. It's acknowledging that you can't raise children alone but need God's intervention. It's also cultivating their relationship with Jesus. **Romans 10;9-10**

As children go to high school, we often feel anxious, wondering how they will survive in a new environment where we have less control over their choices, opinions, and actions. Prayer draws God to action even in your absence. Philippians **4:6-7**. You can concur with me that your parent's prayers have opened doors for your life.

Parenting is warfare because the devil is determined to finish the destinies of our children to eliminate a Godly generation. Prayer destroys every yoke of Satan against our children. No peer influence, drug addiction, fornication, rebellion, and other enemies against our children can survive in the house of a praying parent. Prayer evokes discernment whereby spiritually, you connect with your children, and your spirit reacts when they are in danger.

God aligns the destiny of children through our prayer. No praying parent will raise powerless children. Even when children turn rebellious, call the lord to visit and speak to them. Any spiritual giant is a product of prayer. Let me analyze some biblical examples. Hannah *1 Samuel 1:1-17,* Sarah in *Genesis 21:6-7,* mother of Samson, Elizabeth *Luke 1:25,* Hagar; *Genesis 21:17-17.*

We see these women desperately seeking God's intervention for their children, and GOD answers, and these children become covenant children whom God uses as tools of change. God will grant unto you every desire you have concerning your children. When we don't pray, it's like sitting on the sidelines watching our children in a war zone getting shot from every angle. But prayer means we are beside them in the battle.

## 3.     Kingdom Service

This involves helping your children find their place of service in the house of God. God has packaged gifts for every child, and they require guidance and active involvement.  Let them sing, play instruments, and clean the church, Sunday school, teens department, and youth ministry. Train them on serving with their offerings and strength, serving people, and honoring priests and others. Service roots children in the covenant of Mathew 6:33 (**But seek ye first the kingdom of God, and his righteousness; and all these things shall be added unto you.**)

**Exodus 23:25** *(And ye shall serve the L*ord* your God, and he shall bless thy bread, and thy water, and I will take sickness away from the midst of thee.* The rewards are sure.

Kingdom service launches children in a church system that will help them live exemplary lives. we grew up in church, from Sunday school to youth ministry. This helped us to cultivate our walk in Christ, which rooted our foundation in him.  Today, we are in ministry assisting young people to actualize their dreams because, practically, it has worked for us, and also imparting the same to our children. Therefore, as long as children are under your roof, decide for them by taking them to God; when they grow up, they will prefer to remain in God. Joshua was an example who led the Israelites and told people to choose whichever God they wanted to serve, but for him and his household, he was confident that they would serve the lord. *Joshua 24;14-15*

## 4.      Blessing

Blessings are spiritual influences that affect the spirit of a child to flourish in every circumstance. When God created man, the first things he gave him were blessings to multiply and dominate, influencing their lives. Every man under blessings succeeds. *Psalms 1:1-3* says that blessed people are like trees planted on riverbanks; they never wither, regardless of circumstances. Every child has a glorious, prosperous, Royal and enviable destiny.  And for this to be actualized (*Jeremiah 11:29),* God, as the blesser, has bestowed that responsibility to parents. This involves declaring and speaking positive words over their lives.

The spoken word carries the spirit, which has power for life or death.

*Proverbs 18:21 death and life are in the power of the tongue and they that love it will eat its fruit.*

Therefore, parental words can lock or unlock children's destinies; they go with you wherever you go.

Declarations are sure words of prophesy *Genesis 27; 28-29*. Parents can predict their children's future through declarations and letting them know that they believe God will give them an outstanding life. *Mark 11 says; 23 every word is a seed, and the bible says whatever a man sows, he shall reap. Verse 24:* whatever you desire, you shall receive it. Let your utterance be rooted in scriptures because God's word commits him to manifest. Blessings can turn our children from wickedness and turn their hearts to Jesus *Acts 3:26*. No amount of hard work, seeds, sacrifices, or giving can work in the life of a cursed person.

Biblical examples; -we see God blessing Abraham in *Genesis 12:2-3*. Abraham blessed his son Isaac in *Genesis 26:24,* who prospered in famine until the Egyptians envied him. Isaac also blessed Jacob in **Genesis 27**, who became Israel, God's chosen generation. These blessings made them prosperous.

Contrary to God's will and intent, the devil is always against blessings. As a parent, he may influence you to speak negatively once your children provoke you to stamp a negative influence towards their destiny. This gives him a legal right to attack them; the tongue can rob their destiny. In *Numbers 13:31-33,* we see a story of 10 spies who were sent to spy on the land of Canaan, and a contrary report was brought out that it was impossible to possess the land since the people there were giants and strong. Joshua and Caleb believed they would possess the land in *Numbers 14:6-9.* Once you trace their journey, no Israelite made it to the promised land, only Joshua and Caleb *Numbers 14:30.*

Once you see your life stagnating or falling apart, seek for parental blessings whenever you attempt to progress in marriage, finances, career, ministry, or business. Inculcate in your children the value of parental blessing, and teach them to take advantage of any avenue or channel that can make them get blessed; for example, from spiritual priests, the elderly, giving to the poor, and sharing. This will ensure they succeed without struggle.

**Other Strategies for Effective Parenting.**

## 1. Authority-based parenting.

This kind of parenting portrays parents as the symbol of authority and guidance. Parents place a high demand for achievement and maturity since they are Warm and responsive by teaching their children about morals, values, and goals. They encourage freedom and independence by allowing their kids to handle small tasks as they progress towards heavier duties as they progress in their growth.

They lovingly enforce boundaries by opening up discussions and guiding the children. As a result, these children grow happier, more focused, confident, and independent, have high self-esteem, and are social, not bitter, and insecure.

Whenever the children go against the rules, these parents use alternative disciplinary methods, like confrontative, reasoned, negotiable, outcome-oriented, behavior regulation and modification, and explain their cause of actions. Parents are involved in their children's decisions regarding morals, personal development, performance, self-awareness, career, and peer choice. This is the best parenting strategy since children enjoy the warmth of their parents.

For example, in the Bible, we see King Solomon, who was brought up by an uninvolved parent (King David); we see him being a guide to his son (my son is mentioned 26 times in the book of Proverbs) **Proverbs 1:8, proverbs 23:16-16.** Elkanah and Hannah are also clear examples of those who brought up Samuel in a Godly way and dedicated him to the house of God. He finally became a great prophets under the leadership of Eli, the priest.

Therefore, command sanity in your children. The devil uses worldly systems to entice and influence them to evil patterns. Don't just be calm; this generation is very wild.

## 2. System running parenting.

A system is a set of principles functioning together to achieve a specific goal. Systems are values that guide the behavior of a person. Every company has its systems of running a business, such as integrity, honesty, and fairness, which are clearly defined, and every employee is bound to them.

In this type of parenting, parents adopt a set of procedures and rules to be followed, which is open and engages everyone, creating closeness with the children. If you don't manage your child's behavior when they are young, they will have difficulty learning how to manage themselves when they become older. Any time of the day or night, you should always be able to answer these questions: Where is my child? Who is with my child? What is my child doing? The rules your child has learned from you will shape the rules they will apply.

This system can contain a table of events. Examples include wake-up time, the acceptable code of conduct, when to go to school, prayer and devotion time, playing time, homework time, cartoon and entertainment time. This creates a sort of organized system in their minds. It also boosts their personality in terms of neatness, cleanliness, organization, and social, and brings up an all-round child who can feature in all spheres of life.

Systems also foster your child's independence. Setting limits helps your child develop a sense of self-control. Encouraging independence helps them create a sense of self-direction. To be successful in life, they are going to need both. Remember, it's normal for children to push for autonomy, but many parents mistakenly equate their child's independence with rebelliousness or disobedience.

Children push for independence because it is part of human nature to want to feel in control rather than being controlled. The critical thing here is being consistent. Identify your non-negotiables because if your rules vary from day to day unpredictably, your child's behavior will differ too.

For example, it has taken us over ten years to cultivate a system of prayer and devotion in our house. This entails waking up at 6 am for morning prayers, attending mid-week services, and evening devotion. I knew once a Godly system is instilled in our children's lives, it will regulate their behavior. we realized it was workable when our daughter went to high school and met other girls with immoral behaviors. Her Godly system assisted her in choosing good friends to help her achieve her goals. Even when she comes for holidays, waking up at 6 am for morning devotion has never been a struggle.

This explains why children brought up in well-up financially stable homes may not fit in low-level schools and houses simply because already a standard of living has been set, and that's the system they understand and can cope with. Therefore, identify the system you desire to be instilled in your kids, practice it over time, and it will become part of them. However, a Godly system is the sure way; it will align with all other areas.

## 3. Modeling parenting.
Modeling means learning by observing and copying other people's behavior. Indeed, fruits don't fall far away from the tree. Children are natural mimics. They obey what they observe more than what they are told. A parent is their number one role model, and your actions impact their lives. How often do you see your child imitating your behaviors, like wearing your shoes, wigs, cap, talking, and walking like you? This shows they admire and aspire to be like you. Psychologists say that 80% of children's behaviors are learned through observation. The big question is whether they can learn hard work, diligence, discipline, and acts of kindness from you. Can they emulate your kind of parenting?

This explains why children who grew up in violent and aggressive homes tend to be the same in the future. In relationships and marriage, they turn out to be abusers and batterers. In the bible, the Israelites worshipped other Gods like their fathers did.

*Jeremiah 9:14 (Instead, they have followed the stubbornness of their hearts; they have followed the Baals, as their ancestors taught them."*

How can an alcoholic father warn his children against alcoholism? How do you treat your husband/wife, house manager, or waitress in a restaurant? Your life can inspire or demotivate them, lead or mislead them. Therefore, let them see you pushing hard to make ends meet; it will show them hard work is vital for success.

We dealt with a case where a mother who worked as a barmaid was insecure about her teenage daughter. She couldn't allow her to go out for fear of being tricked by men. During school holidays, she would sit in the house all alone, watching pornography. Being lonely and with sex content in her mind, she resolved to masturbate at a very young age. When she went to college, due to parental modeling, she became a bar lady and a stripper like her mother. Why? Modeling. The big question is, can your children emulate your life?

## 4. Failure v/s achievements parenting.

This means understanding that choices and behaviors have consequences. This is letting your kids learn from your own experiences. Letting your scars teach them the correct route to take. This strategy is best applicable to teenagers who can compromise in life situations. Here, parents don't pose as a "perfect" one; they let them see the roughness of the path and your resilience.

Let us take you down memory lane; remember the mistakes you committed that put you down simply because you lacked guidance or ignorance. The betrayal in that relationship that broke you into pieces, the early pregnancy that made you drop out of school, the drugs that got you expelled to the point you sunken into addiction that affected your investments and wasted your time, it is okey to let them learn through your mistakes and how you fought tearlessly to make it to where you are. Behind every choice and consequence lies a lesson.

If you are in a troubled marriage because of choosing the wrong partner, guide them on the right path to a Godly marriage. Many young people don't believe in marriage simply because they watch their parents struggling, and some come from divorced or unstable homes. A teenage girl confessed that her mother's failures are her motivation simply because she became a single mother of three kids at the age of 24 years. Seeing her struggle single-handedly has steered her motivation to work hard and preserve her life to avoid walking in her mother's shoes.

> *Proverbs 11:21b........................ **but the seed of the righteous shall be delivered.***

The same applies to achievements; always let your achievements motivate them.  A success mentality is cultivated once they see you achieving great milestones. Psalm *112:2-* states that the generation of the upright shall be blessed. It shall strengthen their relationship with God so they can trust his ways to engender generational blessings.

## 5. Attachment strategy replacing fear-based parenting.

Attachment means closeness or warmth. This kind of parenting focuses on strengthening the bond between the parent and a child to nurture the self-worth and emotional well-being of the child.  This strategy helps, mainly when children are grown and portraying negative behaviors like drug addiction and disobedience, especially the youths. However, this strategy works when emotional attachment is maintained from childhood. This is when a parent separates the child from the behavior and tries to see them as God sees them.

Love can change a drug addict. A man we counseled said that when he was in drug addiction, his father chased him from home and denounced him. But her mother dug a hole in the kitchen, put food and a mattress where the boy could come and sleep in the wee hours of the night without the father's knowledge. Her mother could pray for him and tell him he loves him despite his negative behaviors. With time, he overcame, and he confessed that her mother's love, care, and prayers changed him.

Psychologists state that closeness encourages a child to follow instructions and adopt good behaviors. Many youths say it's difficult to confide in their parents on the issues they are facing simply because they feel their parents cannot understand them. This implies a lack of or low attachment.

This strategy replaces the earlier kind of parenting, which was fear-based. Parents then used heavy punishment to instill behavior in children, which worked since that was common to every parent, and children needed to be more informed. The difference comes in when you parent a girl or boy child. Fear-based parenting turns boys to be aggressive, unruly, and disruptive due to the male ego in them. Many are diagnosed with attention deficit disorder, but for girls, it kills their self-worth; therefore, a balance is required to balance the two. Don't spoil or spare the rod either; some behaviors require a rod.

*Proverbs 13:24 whoever spares the rod hates his son, but he who loves him is diligent to discipline him.*

## 6. Exposure parenting strategy.

This kind of parenting subjects' children to new experiences. Statistics show that parental exposure to new experiences increases children's learning outcomes. Exposure brings the hidden to the surface. A child brought up in the village watching their parents' farm cabbages and selling them in the next village market with a donkey cart all his life most probably may amount to do the same. Therefore, let your children visit new places and big hotels, participate in children's activities, and mingle with other children from different backgrounds. This will raise the level of their ambitions and desire to achieve more.  One day, our daughter saw a girl in her early twenties driving a pink car; it motivated her to work hard and drive the same at a young age.

Exposure widens the information in the mental base, hence creating more ideas. Psychologists state that events, situations, and environments shape a behavior's perception, attitude, and motivation. For example, in the parliament buildings of Kenya, We often see students visiting in large numbers. This stirs up inspiration and motivation to be great leaders who serve our country. Exposure should be limited to what is beneficial to children.

This applies to harmful exposure to wrong information. It has a way of empowering the mental faculties to act. For example, exposure to sexual content at an early age creates curiosity in children, and they end up practicing the same. Let the level of positive exposure be beyond their level now.

This is a game changer in parenting and shapes the behavior and aspirations of children. Let your children be restricted to the home environment because allowing them to loiter around will expose them to negative influences. We often see school-going children asking for free rides from personal cars and motorbikes. Many have fallen victim to abuse and kidnappings. Exposure empowers imagination and action.

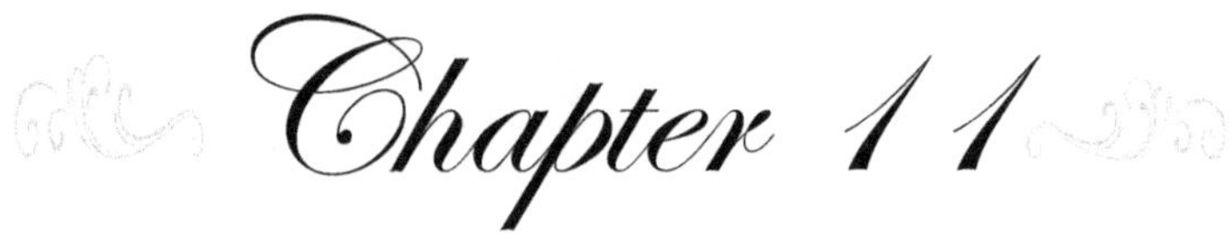

# Chapter 11

## Mistakes Parents Commit Against Children.

Parents have a unique way of bringing up children, but they are prone to mistakes that they don't realize in their journey. The truth is that everyone faces different challenges when growing up, which makes some children flourish and become well-adjusted adults while others may not be so blessed with ideal conditions. The biggest mistake parents can make is underestimating their ongoing influence or impact on their children.

Some parents have no idea, while others think this effect disappears after children reach a certain age. But the truth is, it doesn't; they carry the impact throughout their lifetime. So here are some common parenting mistakes that negatively affect children's growth. These mistakes may be favorable to parents, but trust me; they affect our children big time.

## 1. Abuse or Toxicity.

Abuse refers to an act of treatment with cruelty or violence, especially regularly or repeatedly. In the Bible, all violence is considered an offense against God and humanity. Also, Jesus tells us that the kingdom of God is like a little child, and whatsoever we do to the least of these, we do to him.
Abuse in parenting is portrayed by physical injuries, Verbal abuse (yelling, name-calling, threatening, manipulating, and criticizing), Emotional abuse, neglect, and financial neglect.

Any form of abuse leaves visible and invisible scars since it leaves the victim feeling like a shell of a person, separated from the true essence of who they naturally are. It also leads to a victim feeling tormented and tortured by their own emotions and identity. Many end up being anti-social and have difficulty in relationships with others.
The Bible prohibits this in *Ephesians 6:4 And, ye fathers, provoke not your children to wrath: but bring them up in the nurture and admonition of the Lord.*

God approves discipline but not in excessive. Out of ten counseling sessions that we handle, 8 cases are primarily caused by childhood abuse, especially verbal and emotional abuse.

*Colossians 3:21Fathers, provoke not your children to anger, lest they be discouraged.*

Provocation breeds discouragement and failure. Using humiliation, especially in front of their friends, as discipline leads to embarrassment, behavioral and emotional problems in the future - many end up being socially anxious, depressed, or aggressive.

**2. Comparing your children to others in terms of performance and behavior.**

This ruins a child's early self-esteem and makes them question their parents' love. A client said this to us:" My mom used to compare me with other children all the time. And when I had a confrontation with any other kid, she'd always take their side. So, I grew up with a mentality that my mom loved other kids more than me. Eventually, I stopped telling her about my problems, whenever i was bullied or had a conflict with the teacher. All she would say was, "It was your fault." I'm 23years now, and I still have enormous difficulties with sharing my problems with anyone."

Therefore, when you compare your child with their friends, brothers, or sisters in terms of behavior or performance, it covers them with a cloud of confusion and they tend to think that they are living below your expectations. Many try to please you as a parent, and once they realize you are not noticing, they give up, which ruins their motivation and confidence.  When they grow up, these children tend to do things to please others to gain favor and acceptance even at the expense of their lives which the bible condemns in

*Galatians 1:10 (For am I now seeking the approval of man or God? Or am I trying to please man? If I were still trying to please man, I would not be a servant [of Christ.)*

This results in demotivation, and since they lack the willpower, they must always be pushed to achieve in life. Once employed, they give their supervisors a lot of work because they can't work under minimum supervision and many end up being sacked. The same applies to grades; children possess different intellectual capabilities. Whether one child is performing better than the other, it should not breed comparisons.

Every child is unique, and comparison is termed as lack of wisdom and understanding.

*2 Corinthians 10:12 (Not that we dare to classify or compare ourselves with some of those who are commending themselves. But when they measure themselves by one another and compare themselves with one another, they are without understanding.)*

## 3. Negative or positive Parental Negligence.

Every child desires to be brought up by both parents because it stabilizes the child's development. Damaging negligence comes when parents deny children security, basic needs, love, happiness, acceptance, and stability. Children don't need an extravagant life, but they want to see parents trying hard to fight for their welfare, and despite their financial status, there is joy, peace, sacrifice, love, and goodwill.

A client confessed that he blames his father for not educating him, and he was financially able.

*Psalms 27:10(Though my father and mother forsake me, the LORD will receive me.)*

But even if God proves to be the only source of refuge, creating parenting gaps is termed as negligence.

In brief, let's address the issue of children born out of wedlock and abandoned at the grandmother's place.
A certain lady narrated her upbringing journey to us. She was taken to her grandmother's home at the age of 7

months, and the mother went to Nairobi and got married. After two years, the grandmother was overburdened by responsibilities and took her back to her mother who was pregnant by then like a parcel in a matatu.

This began a journey of turmoil because her mother called her cursed and an obstacle to her ambition, and her stepdad treated her as an outcast. After a traumatic upbringing, the identity crisis fueled her to look for her biological dad since she felt neglected, but the efforts didn't bear fruits. She is 37 years now but the effects of rejection are still in her life. She faces this spirit of rejection everywhere from work place, family members, church, and friends to the point even her marriage dissolved. After we walked through a journey of self –acceptance and prayed against rejection, her life changed. She is now reunited with her husband, family members and trauma-free.

Parental negligence might result from a positive reason, such as work demands, whereby many travel far to work, leaving their children under the care of relatives. For parents, I agree it's for a worthy cause, but not for children. Children feel neglected and substituted for work and money. This affects their closeness with their parents even if they are provided with the best life.

Our friend, who was brought up by her grandmother, told us that she began addressing her real mother as "mum" at the age of 20 years since she was far working, and all along, she knew her grandmother as her mother. Today, she is married and has children, and it is easier to confide in her grandmother when she needs guidance than the mother.

## 4. Involving children in conflicts and disagreements.

Any disagreements between parents affect the children. These conflicts emerging from marital conflicts and divorces affect the children more. Conflicts corrupt the atmosphere physically, emotionally, and mentally. A stable family is protected under a spiritual force around it; the hedge of protection repels the enemy, as in the case of Job.

**Job 1:10.** Conflicts break the hedge and expose children to satanic attacks.

*Ecclesiastes 10:8 He that diggeth a pit shall fall into it; and whoever breaketh a hedge, a serpent shall bite him.*

The effects of conflicts like war, abuse, wasted resources, and emotional turmoil hits children directly. Many have resolved to bitterness and running away from home to escape the Vietnam War zone at home. And while looking for safety and peace, many end up falling into the wrong hands. A 13-year-old girl in one high school said that she was impregnated by a man she ran to after escaping from a chaotic environment where mum and dad always fought every night. These fights had impacted a lot of fear in her and her siblings, to the point they developed academic problems, depression, panic attacks, fear, and anxiety.

Conflicts also impact a negative mindset in children where the Majority end up having poor marriages and relationships in the future due to poor modeling. Therefore, despite disagreements, always think of the primary victims. Your children should never and will never be put in between your conflicts. It will do more harm than good, which is unfair to them.

## 5. Favoritism

This implies having a favorite, which is evident when a parent gives one child more love, attention, favor, and affirmation over the other. This mostly happens when one child performs better than the other.

**Genesis 25:28** highlights the story of Esau and Jacob, in which the parents played one's favorite. Isaac loved Esau, but Rebecca loved Jacob. This stirred his mother to incite his second-born son Jacob to lie against his father to receive firstborn blessings. This caused hatred.

**Genesis 37:3-4** records a story of Joseph, who was loved more by his father, Jacob, than by his brothers. This became a generational spirit since Jacob replicated the same spirit of favoritism to his child, just as his mother did to him—this caused jealousy, which resulted to him being sold into slavery by his brothers.

This is common in our daily life, with brothers and sisters stating categorically that their mother loves some children more and the father the same. I saw a family fighting against their sister simply because they believed their father loved her and educated her more than. The irony is the brothers were more successful career-wise than the sister. Up to date, they are reluctant to help her establish herself. I heard one brother say," Let her father help her. After all, he used all her retirement benefits to educate her".

This might have been true or untrue to parents; children pick up some actions parents do and interpret how they deem fit. This calls for balance, especially regarding privileges, rewards, favors, and compliments.

## 6.	Being over-protective

In earlier times, parenting was harsh, and children were exposed to challenging and demanding situations, which made them mature and responsible at a tender age. Children could take care of cattle in large grazing fields as early as eight years old and sometimes encounter wild animals. And by evening, they would return home with the meat they had hunted from the fields. These hardships were not easy, but they helped children to be thinkers and solution-oriented.

Today, an 8-year-old boy can scream at the sight of a chicken being slaughtered. Why? Every parent desires to give their children a simpler life free from the difficulties they encounter. Insecurities brought by failures they encountered have served as a motivation to shield their children from failure and harm. As a result, children are brought up tender like a yolk in an eggshell.

This is when parents protect their children from failure and disappointment, even if it means going against the law. They control their children's actions, including making decisions for them, creating a sense of dependency. When these children grow up and face the world, demanding systems threaten them, and they surrender and give in to various vices.

Children should be allowed to make mistakes and fail sometimes and be guided on re-correcting. Over-protection raises a mentally weak generation with low coping mechanisms; they avoid interactions, pressures, and conflicts, and when they face them, they can easily crumble.

This is the reason behind raising half-baked men who have no authority in their homes, especially with the empowered girl child. It's not a wonder to see a woman looking for money and feeding the man all her life simply because he lost his job or he is out drinking alcohol. This is unacceptable. Despite difficulties, as a man, you must do what you can to feed your family and maintain respect and authority.

Over-protection makes it difficult for some parents to release their children even after marriage due to fear of them facing challenges. This makes them interfere with their son's or daughters' marriages in terms of decision-making to shield them from any marital pressure. Once a conflict arises, they hurriedly advise their daughters to return home. This shows low resilience in solving problems that can destroy their lives.

## 7. Financial Dependency on Their Children.

A child is supposed to enjoy parental financial cover until they attain an age of independence, especially after college or university and getting into the job market. But today, the case is reversed: once parents educate the firstborn and second born, once they step into the job market earning peanuts, they are given responsibilities to educating the other siblings. And instead of allowing them to continue upgrading their lives, this responsibility cripples their financial destiny. Others are tasked with the burden of buying land and building for their parents to remove them from shame and despair. Others depend on their children for basic needs like food, clothing, and shelter.

I don't refute that it's a blessing for children to assist their parents, but it should be out of the will to honor and appreciate them. The sad thing is that their parents relax once these children take up this responsibility. Amid children fighting through life to provide for themselves, they are forced to engage in risky behaviors like prostitution and selling drugs since responsibilities are too many compared to whatever they are earning. As parents, let us plan and create a retirement plan for ourselves.

It is even anti-God if we are waiting for our now 6-year-old girl to help us in life. We are supposed to take her to university and give her a footstool for inheritance to push her life. Once they mature and become independent, if they decide to upgrade their parent's life at an old age, it is purely their decision.

The Bible states in **Proverbs13:22**; *that a Good man leaves an inheritance to their grandchildren, including financial inheritance.*

A man claimed that he stagnated financially and could not educate his children to college since he assumed all his father's responsibilities to educate their siblings. It also broke his marriage due to financial constraints. For this man, it's unfair to him and his family. That is why many parents have lost honor and respect for their children. A lady told me that he barely talks with his father since every time he demands money from her, and if she doesn't send it, her father rebukes her and curses her. But the truth is those curses are empty because the parents are bestowed with responsibility for their children, not vice versa. Even children go the extra mile to pay the dowry for their mother on behalf of their father. Even in the traditional culture, this is wrong.

Unless extreme and exceptional cases are understandable, mainly due to parental sickness or calamities. But if the parent is in good shape, work extra hard to offset these burdens from your children. It damages their lives and families, too.

## 8. Giving inheritance with conditions.
As I said earlier, assets are vital to every child for a startup. The problem sets in when parents attach conditions to these assets. This invokes a curse upon them once they go contrary. Many parents especially give their children land with conditions that they should not sell.

We have seen children lavishing in poverty with a title of 10 acres in a prime area worth millions. Exceptional cases are understandable, especially where children are deep in drugs and alcohol.

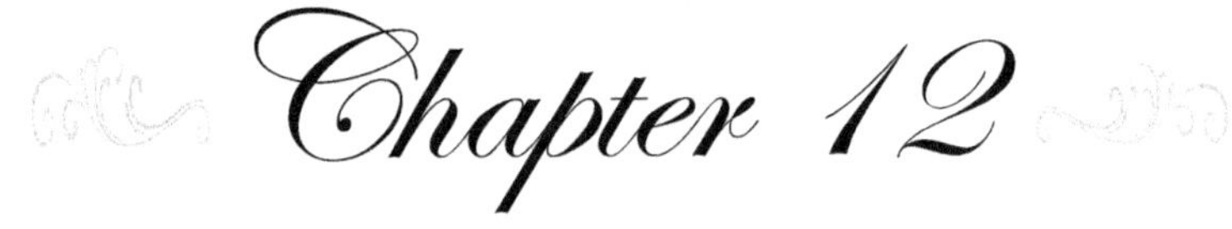

# Chapter 12

## EPILOGUE.

The success of a parenting journey is not only measured by how children achieve professionally or career-wise but also by who they become and how they view God, themselves, and others. The big question is, have you led them through a journey of self-actualization? Children who can serve God, themselves, and humanity? Children who are agents of change in organizations, companies, and the world? Therefore, if your influence and connection are carried over by your children even in your absence, this is successful parenting.

*2Corinthians 6:18 And will be a Father unto you, and ye shall be my sons and daughters, saith the Lord Almighty,*

This scripture portrays God as our father; hence, he demands that we replicate God's parenting to our children. The word of God is plain on children and promises a glorious destiny for them. Therefore, even when children portray negative behavior contrary to your expectations declare the word of God upon them and focus on the journey.

When you see failure, declares Isaiah 8:18: *Behold I and the children the LORD has given me. We are signs and symbols in Israel from the LORD Almighty, who dwells on Mount Zion.*

When the devil brings darkness and confusion, declare light and order upon them.
*Matthew 5:14 you are the light of the world. A town built on a hill cannot be hidden.*

Once you see their destiny crumble, declare Deuteronomy 28:13: *And the LORD shall make thee the head, and not the tail; and thou shalt be above only, and thou shalt not be beneath,* and God is quick and faithful to obey his word in favor of your children.

And after the journey, a crown or prize is sure, and you will indeed say

*2 Timothy 4:7 I have fought a good fight, I have finished my course, I have kept the faith: henceforth there is laid up for me a crown of righteousness, which the Lord, the righteous judge, shall give me at that day: and not to me only, but unto all them also that love his appearing.*

Remember, parenting is in seasons. When **you are in** control of your children, when they are under *their* control, and when **you are under** their care (old age). Enjoy every season by investing wisely because their treatment will be determined by how you treat them. If you planted seeds of hate, arrogance, and rebellion, they will abandon you to rot in the village, and your labor will be a waste. Let them desire your God and your parenting strategy. They will understand and accomplish their God-given purpose when equipped with Godly values. Their obedience to God's instructions will make their family work. When a family works, the body of Christ will be intact, and it will shed light on the whole world.

The bottom line is that if your children live under criticism, they learn to condemn. If they live in a hostile environment, they learn how to fight. If they live under tolerance, they learn patience. If they live with encouragement, they learn to be confident. If they live under praise, they learn to appreciate others. If they live under fairness, they learn justice. If they live under approval, they learn how to love themselves. If they live under acceptance and friendship, they learn to find love in the world. This is intentional parenting.

## PRAYER.

Our prayer is that none of you will reap tears. we declare that your children shall not fail in your hands. Your labor will not be in vain. The grace of Godly parenting will be replicated in your life; you shall reap the fruits of your labor. You shall not die until you see the Lord bless and uplift your children. They will serve the lord all the days of their life. Their destinies are secured and favored upon their careers, health, visions, and aspirations.  Your generation is preserved in Jesus' name.

## References


1. "The Collapse of Parenting: *How We Hurt Our Kids When We Treat Them Like Grown-Ups*" by Leonard Sax, MD, PhD

2. "The Blessing of a Skinned Knee: *Using Jewish Teachings to Raise Self-Reliant Children*" by Wendy Mogel, PhD

3. "The Price of Privilege: *How Parental Pressure and Material Advantage Are Creating a Generation of Disconnected and Unhappy Kids*" by Madeline Levine, PhD

4. "The Coddling of the American Mind: *How Good Intentions and Bad Ideas Are Setting Up a Generation for Failure*" by Greg Lukianoff and Jonathan Haidt

5. "Parenting in the Age of Attention Snatchers: *A Step-by-Step Guide to Balancing Your Child's Use of Technology*" by Lucy Jo Palladino, PhD

Epilogue.

Epilogue.